THE DIVINELY RESPONDING CLASSIC

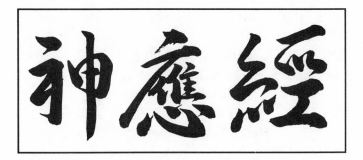

The Divinely
Responding Classic

A Translation of the *Shen Ying Jing* from the *Zhen Jiu Da Cheng*

translated by
Yang Shou-zhong
and Liu Feng-ting

BLUE POPPY PRESS

Published by:

BLUE POPPY PRESS
1775 LINDEN AVE.
BOULDER, CO 80304

First Edition, September, 1994

ISBN 0-936185-55-4
LC 93-74979

COMP Designation: Denotative translation

Printed at Westview Press, Boulder, CO on acid free, recycled paper. Cover
Printed at C&M Press, Thornton, CO.
Cover portrait by Wang Yong-xing and Sun Shu-wen
Cover calligraphy by Michael Sullivan (Seiho)

recycled paper

10 9 8 7 6 5 4 3 2

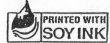

Translator's Preface

T his book is a denotative translation of the eighth book or treatment formulary section of the *Zhen Jiu Da Cheng (Great Compendium of Acupuncture & Moxibustion)* compiled by Yang Ji-zhou in the late Ming dynasty as found in the People's Health and Hygiene Press, Beijing, 1983 edition and excepting the discrepancies discussed below.

As is well known, the foundations of Traditional Chinese Medicine (TCM) and acupuncture/moxibustion were laid by the beginning of the Han dynasty. All the seminal theories of this system of healing are available in the *Su Wen (Simple Questions)*, the *Ling Shu (Spiritual Pivot)*, and the *Nan Jing (Classic of Difficulties)*. Nonetheless, since the Han, TCM and acupuncture have never stopped growing, and practitioners and scholars in each past historical period have contributed something to this lore. However, the most intellectually fecund period for the growth of TCM theory and practice was the Jin/Yuan dynasties (1115-1368 CE). This is because of a number of factors, not least of which was the development of Neoconfucianism and the intellectual ferment this movement produced. I have discussed these factors at some length in my preface to the Li Dong-yuan's *Pi Wei Lun (Treatise on the Spleen & Stomach)* also published by Blue Poppy Press as part of their Great Masters Series.

The fact that the Jin/Yuan dynasties were an especially prolific period in the development of Chinese medical practices and theories does not mean that, as some contemporary Chinese historians have asserted, nothing of much importance happened in the theoretical development of Chinese medicine between the end of the Han and the beginning of the Jin/Yuan dynasties. Hua Tuo (*circa* 110-207 CE) and Zhang Zhong-jing (*circa* 150-219 CE) are everlasting credits to TCM who lived in the late Han dynasty, while the Tang dynasty boasted Sun Si-miao (*circa* 581-682 CE) who has been enshrined as a medical god. However, these outstanding medical personages appeared like separate stars, while in the Jin/Yuan dynasties, TCM was illuminated by a bright galaxy. This bright galaxy of TCM luminaries was none other than the four great masters surrounded by their numerous accomplished disciples, and their prolific thinking and research efforts were beams of light radiating in every direction of TCM.

Likewise, acupuncture and moxibustion have enjoyed a similar crowning glory which came soon after the Jin/Yuan period, during the Ming dynasty (1368-1644 CE). The most celebrated of celebrated scholar-acupuncturists of that time was Yang Ji-zhou (1522-1620 CE), styled Ji-shi (Benefitting the World), the author of the *Zhen Jiu Da Cheng*. He was born into a medical family. His grandfather was a physician in the then imperial medical academy and was very much in favor with the emperor. This notwithstanding, Yang Ji-zhou did not at first choose medicine as his future career. He followed a path trod by many distinguished TCM physicians in ancient times, first learning the Confucian classics as preparation for entrance into officialdom. Such study resulted in these would-be scholar-officials becoming well versed in many branches of the humanities. However, like a number of other famous Chinese doctors of antiquity, Yang turned to the study of medicine after failing the examinations for the Confucian imperial bureaucracy. As a youth, Yang was a talented student, and, while still quite young, he, in fact, passed the official examination as a promising candidate for a government position. However, because the official examiner in his region was prejudiced against him, his ambition to become an official was thwarted. He then became determined to "benefit the world" by means of medicine.

Responding Classic) by Liu Jin, the *Zhen Jiu Ju Ying (Gatherings from Outstanding Acupuncture/Moxibustion Works)* by Gao Wu from 1529, the *Gu Jin Yi Tong Da Quan (Comprehensive Collection of Medical Works Past & Present)* by Xu Chun-fu from 1556, the *Zhen Jiu Jie Yao (Acupuncture/Moxibustion Excerpts from the Classics)* by Gao Wu, the *Zhen Jiu Wen Dui (Questions & Answers on Acupuncture & Moxibustion)* by Wang Ji from 1530, the *Yi Xue Ru Men (Entering the Gate of the Study of Medicine)* by Li Yan from 1575, etc. All of these are acclaimed, authoritative works in this field, and all of them were achievements of the Ming dynasty. These works formed a fertile soil, and fertile soil must produce a bountiful crop. By now everything necessary for the birth of a great classic was ready. At last, in 1601 CE, it was given to the world.

The *Zhen Jiu Da Cheng* consists of ten books. It is a *magnum opus* both in terms of quality and quantity. The first book consists of discussions of the theories of acumoxatherapy drawn from the *Nei Jing (Inner Classic)*, the *Ling Shu*, and the *Nan Jing*. The second and third books are a collection of all the important poems and rhymes for the study and memorization of this art available up to that time. The composing of rhymes and songs as mnemonic devices teaching beginners the rudimentary facts of acupuncture and moxibustion was a common practice in the Yuan and Ming dynasties. The fourth book contains discussions by outstanding medical figures, including Yang Ji-zhou himself, about the various needling manipulations and especially those concerning supplementation and drainage. Book five is about the *zi wu liu zhu liao fa* or midnight-midday point selection method. The next two books are treatises on the viscera and bowels, channels and connecting vessels, and acupoints. The eighth book, which has been translated herein, is a compendium of acupuncture and moxibustion formulas for the treatment of various diseases. Book nine is a collection of the peculiar needling and moxaing treatment methods invented by earlier outstanding TCM scholars and physicians. The last book is about pediatric *tui na*, *i.e.*, remedial massage for the treatment of children.

Ever since its birth, this work has been universally acknowledged as the most authoritative and mature in the premodern literature of acupuncture and moxibustion. Even until now, no other work can be said to truly challenge either its theoretical or practical value. Looking back at the history of this art, the *Su Wen* and *Ling Shu*, and particularly the latter, are its foundation. The *Huang Di Zhen Jiu Jia Yi Jing (Yellow Emperor's Systematic Classic of Acupuncture & Moxibustion)* created its basic framework. The *Zhen Jiu Da Cheng* completed the building and ornamentation of this great treasure house.

These are the three milestones in the Chinese evolution of the art of acupuncture and moxibustion. The words *da cheng* to a Chinese mean the ultimate completion of a great work, the consummate understanding of all relevant branches of a science, and an all-embracing collection. This work deserves that title. An interesting fact shows how it has been valued, how influential it has been, and how widely it has been circulated. In 1657, only 56 years after its first publication, its second edition was printed. Then 23 years later, a third edition came out. Then another 56 years and a fourth version was brought out. During the Qing dynasty (1644-1911 CE), 28 editions of the *Zhen Jiu Da Cheng* were published. During those times, printing was extremely expensive and labor-intensive, let alone printing such a voluminous work. Rarely did a premodern work, no matter what it was, enjoy such a privilege if it was not truly exceptional. Before Liberation, *i.e.*, from 1911-1949, 14 editions were added to this list. In other words, during that period, a new edition of the *Da Cheng* was published at an average of every 6.8 years! Even now when we have the unrivaled advantage of computerized printing equipment, how many other 300 year old books receive a new edition every 6.8 years?

Yang's source for the eighth book of the *Zhen Jiu Da Cheng*, the most clinically significant section of this compendium, is mainly the *Shen Ying Jing* or *Divinely Responding Classic* mentioned above. The fact that Yang Ji-zhou chose this work as the basis of his treatment formulary section demonstrates how highly he held this work. The *Shen Ying Jing* was originally compiled by Liu Jin who, in turn, based it on the *Guan Ai Shu (Book of Universal Love)* by his master, Chen Hong-gang. In the process of compiling the *Zhen Jiu Da Cheng*, Yang Ji-zhou edited the *Shen Ying Jing*, dividing it into parts, rearranging these parts in different books, modifying its text in a small number of places, and omitting some paragraphs. In preparing this current volume, we have endeavored to the best of our ability to restore the original form of the *Shen Jing Ying* so that it can stand on its own, both as an historical source and as a useful clinical manual. In any case, there is only a little difference between the version of the *Shen Ying Jing* as it appears herein and its counterpart in the eighth book of the *Zhen Jiu Da Cheng*. The exception to this statement is that we have chosen not to include the section on point locations and indications. This material has already been incorporated into English language texts, such as O'Connor & Bensky's *Acupuncture: A Comprehensive Text* and Ellis, Wiseman & Boss' *Fundamentals of Chinese Acupuncture*.

On the other hand, besides the *Shen Ying Jing*, the *Zhen Jiu Da Cheng* includes some materials from other sources in the eighth book. In order to present the English-speaking acupuncture community a version conducive to clinical practice and academically authentic, while restoring the original look of the *Shen Ying Jing*, I have also preserved all these materials added by Yang Ji-zhou outside the *Shen Ying Jing*. These are found at the back of the current text as in the eighth book of the *Da Cheng*. They are clearly identifiable by the author's original notations before each such part. In other words, the translator has not made any changes to the eighth book of the *Zhen Jiu Da Cheng* except for the restoration of the parts of the *Shen Ying Jing* relegated by

Yang Ji-zhou to other books within the *Da Cheng* and the omission of the section on point locations and indications. This accounts for the reason why we have added a subtitle to this translation.

The terminology and methodology used in this translation are based upon Nigel Wiseman and Ken Boss' *Glossary of Chinese Medical Terms and Acupuncture Points*. In regard to the point names, it is the genuine belief of the translator that Wiseman and Boss' *Glossary*, in general, advances a more credible and more accurately defined set of terms than any other work of its kind to which he has had access, including those that are designed by Chinese scholars in the People's Republic of China in recent years. In all probability, its success lies in its compilers being not biased towards any one school but having absorbed nearly all the reasonable approaches contained in the various relevant reference materials available to them. However, as the understanding of the meanings of the various point names has always been rather a controversial issue, no one can come up with a design that will be universally acknowledged without any error.

In the *Glossary*, a small number of the point names are, it seems to the translator, open to discussion. For one thing, we favor a uniform treatment of the same Chinese character, even if only out of consideration for facilitating the memorization of the English speaking learner, in so far as the English translation causes no misunderstanding. Take *fu* (府) as an example. We believe it is not necessary to translate this single character by so many variants of mansion, abode, storehouse, treasury, etc., as in the *Glossary*. At least we would reduce the number. However, in connection with such point names, we have followed Wiseman *et al.*'s lead lest we create even more confusion than convenience.

xii

We also feel that the authors of the *Glossary* have failed to correctly convey the meanings of some point names. For *Gong Sun* (Sp 4), it gives "Yellow Emperor." According to certain sources, the surname of the Yellow Emperor was possibly, but only possibly, Gong Sun. (In fact, most historians say his surname was Ji.) Assuming his name to be Gong Sun, the Yellow Emperor has never simply been called this in any Chinese literature but is most frequently addressed as Huang, Xuan, or Xuan Yuan Shi. The Yellow Emperor was worshipped as a god and using his surname directly would have been deemed blasphemous and quite against Chinese cultural tradition. What is more important, we cannot find another example of naming a point after a great person throughout the whole system of Chinese acupoint nomenclature.

Ling Xu (Ki 24), which is rendered as "Spirit Ruins" in the *Glossary*, seems to us to be another example of misinterpretation. *Xu* may mean ruins, but equally possibly, village or countryside. Its alternative name, *Ling Qiang*, clears the ambiguity. *Qiang* in Chinese is defined as none other than wall. Furthermore, based on the Chinese concepts of omens and coincidence, it obviously would have been improper to name a remedy ruins. On that account, we would prefer such translations as Spirit Village or Spirit Homeland.

In any case, the English point names we consider unacceptable in the *Glossary* are only a handful in number. In preparing this book, we have abandoned them and have adopted our own coinings. They include *Pu Can* (Bl 61, Subservient Visitor: Servant Kneeling), *Tong Li* (Ht 5, Connecting *Li*: Connecting the Interior), *Zhang Men* (Liv 13, Camphorwood Gate: Screen Gate), and *Da Zhui* (GV 14, Great Hammer: Great Vertebra) besides *Gong Sun* (Sp 4, Yellow Emperor: Offspring of the Noble) and *Ling Xu* (Ki 24, Spirit Ruins: Spirit Homeland). We have also changed Kunlun Mountains (*Kun Lun*, Bl 60) to Kunlun (Mountain). In China, there are two different mountains called Kunlun.

One is the chain of mountains north of Tibet. The other is the solitary mountain known in Angelicized Sanskrit as Kailash. Since this point lies behind the medial malleolus which stands up alone like the great Mt. Kailash, we believe this point is named after it rather than the Kunlun range of mountains. There are yet some other point names we do not completely agree with Wiseman *et al.* concerning their English renditions. However, theirs are acceptable nevertheless. Again, for fear of creating confusion, we have complied with them despite our disagreement.

In this book, acupoints are identified first by the English translation of their name. This is then followed in parentheses by the *Pinyin* spelling of their name, a comma, and a numerical identification based on the number of points located on each channel, ergo: Screen Gate (*Zhang Men,* Liv 13). These numerical identifications are based on the World Health Organization's *Proposed Standard International Acupuncture Nomenclature* (WHO, Geneva, 1991) except for the following discrepancies: For the lung channel, we use Lu instead of LU; for the stomach, we use St instead of ST; for the spleen, we use Sp instead of SP; for the heart, we use Ht instead of HT; for the bladder, we use Bl instead of BL; for the kidney, we use Ki instead of KI; for the pericardium, we use Per instead of PC; for the triple heater, we use TH instead of TE; and for the liver, we use Liv instead of LR. Identifications of extra-channel points are based on the numbering system in O'Connor & Bensky's *Acupuncture: A Comprehensive Text* published by Eastland Press.

Materials appearing in brackets have been added by unknown Chinese editors and appear in the Chinese edition upon which this translation has been based. Materials appearing in parentheses have been added by the translator to clarify and to make the text sound better in English.

Yang Shou-zhong
Tangshan, Hebei, PRC

(Han Xi-ji's) Preface
to the Second (Chinese) Edition
of the *Shen Ying Jing*

I n the sixth year after ascending to the palace, His Respectable Majesty issued a decree to the Ministry of Honor instructing it to carry out more vigorous medical education. (In addition,) the Medical Learning Institute (was instructed) to establish a special program for acupuncture and moxibustion. The best in the art were to be selected as the masters and bright and intelligent (youths) as (their) protégés. It (also) stipulated elaborately detailed regulations for encouragement (of this art) and incentives (for its practice and propagation).

At that time, it so happened that a Japanese Buddhist Ryoshin came to present the *Shen Ying Jing* and, simultaneously, to impart an eight point treatment protocol for *yong* and *ju* invented by his fellow countrymen, the divine physicians Wasuke and Niba. Although these eight points had never been tried and practiced, the teaching of the *Shen Ying Jing* had had a long history (in China. This book) illustrates a (point) locating method and supplementing and draining manipulations which ancient sages had not shed light upon. In many places, its point selection reveals the negligence of the ancients. The points included in it are all essential and crucial ones that are effective in a vast range of diseases. Its language being concise, this work is filled with an all-inclusive content. Thus its readers are able to get a clear picture before their eyes about the signs and points (to be chosen) after perusing it (for only) a little while. Therefore, His Majesty exclaimed in praise, ordering to print the *Shen Ying Jing* with the eight point method as an appendix put at the back in hope that it would circulate widely and pass down to infinite future.

My humble self bethinks that, in terms of medical therapies, neither medication nor acumoxatherapy should be favored at one another's expense. (However,) among medicinals there are many which are not homegrown. In general, people are supposed to seek medicinals in China, but, in fact, they are not all China's produce. (Sometimes, therefore,) one has to trade or purchase them in a rather roundabout way. Apart from the difficulty of obtaining them, there is often no choosing between the genuine and fake or between the fresh and stale. Besides, the poor and humble and those living in remote places hardly have access to (such medicinals). On the contrary, the therapy of the stone needle and moxibustion may rid one of the expense (of buying medicinals), the trouble of having to seek them from far away, and the difficulty of gathering, drying, and mixing them. Needles and moxa, which are all that are required and which need no particular formula (to be prepared in advance), are operated with but the fingers, (and the treatment) is accomplished amidst chats and jokes. It is inappropriate to none, neither the poor nor the rich, neither the noble nor the humble, neither those living near nor those living far off, neither the urgent nor the mild (problems). In addition, very often it brings effect to the places from which the attack launched that the strength of medicinals falls short of. It is hardly possible to give an exhaustive account of (all) its wonderful uses. Vulgar physicians are ignorant, assuming (acupuncture/moxibustion) as a base and humiliating (art), thus discrediting it, and will not apply it to the sick. As a result, the sick in the world have to trust their life and death, their longevity and premature death to witchery, incantation, and religious performance. Is this not lamentable!

His Majesty, taking pity on this situation, introduced a special institution (for the research and teaching of acupuncture and

Because his family owned myriads of medical books and, moreover, because he was very intelligent, as well as diligent, it took him only a short time to become perfectly proficient in TCM theory and practice. Soon his reputation of having two magical hands that could instantly bring spring even to a dead person spread across the country. Later he was several times invited to serve the sick in the royal family. Yang Ji-zhou held a position as a physician in the imperial palace for many years.

Long before that, however, he had begun to cherish a wish to gather all the important works on acupuncture and moxibustion together and publish them in a collection. In ancient China, few, if any, physicians were rich enough to raise the funds sufficient to accomplish such an end. In his youth, Yang once had tried to publish a book much thinner than what he was now planning. It was called the *Wei Sheng Xuan Ji Mi Yao (Life-defending Secret Essentials of the Mysterious Mechanisms [of Acupuncture & Moxibustion])*. This manuscript had been in his family's possession possibly for many generations, but his effort had ended in failure because of financial problems. It should be remembered that there were no private publishing houses which published books for profit. Authors had to publish books out of their own pockets or else find a wealthy patron.

Besides, Yang had another difficulty in realizing his aspiration. A single family's collection, even if it were large, was not sufficient to stand as a book on its own. And at that time, acquiring books, most which were still hand copied and handed down from teacher to student, was no easy task. It happened that a provincial governor, Zhao Wen-bing, was bed-ridden with chronic atony bordering on paralysis. Zhao was a very important man of his time. He invited Yang Ji-zhou for a treatment after having consulted a great many other physicians of various sorts in vain. As in a myth, only three acupuncture treatments brought spring back! The governor felt deeply indebted besides being amazed at Yang Ji-zhou's marvelous skill. Therefore, he

vii

readily promised to help turn Yang's lifelong dream into a reality with his financial backing, retainers, and political power.

As mentioned above, in the Ming dynasty and especially toward its end, acupuncture and moxibustion enjoyed a brilliant crescendo in China. This was first because the emperors of that dynasty gave great importance to this art. It was a Ming emperor who ordered to rebuild a standard acupuncture bronze statue to replace the one cast in the Song dynasty. This had stood for more than 400 years. It was also a Ming emperor that proposed renewing the stone carving of the *Tong Ren Shu Xue Zhen Jiu Tu Jing (Acupuncture & Moxibustion Classic of the Atlas of the Points on the Bronze Man)*. Those wishing to study acupuncture and moxibustion could take rubbings from these carvings, thus learning the standard names and locations of the channels and their points. In a time when books were scarce and hard to come by, establishing such public access was a great boon to the popularization and propagation of this art. This was an event of tremendous historical significance. During imperial times, the predilections of the emperor were certain to have a decisive bearing upon any field they chose to show their favor.

In addition, the flourishing of acumoxatherapy in this period was the result of the accretion and evolution of this art over its long history. Towards the late Ming dynasty, acupuncture and moxibustion developed to such a height that each and every branch of the study, from its theories of the channels and connecting vessels to its needling manipulations, had become mature and had reached a consummate level. From this point of view, the flourishing of acupuncture and moxibustion during this period was but the fruition and harvesting of many centuries of slow growth and development.

In a preface to an early, authoritative edition of the *Zhen Jiu Da Cheng*, the author of the preface lists the materials Yang Ji-zhou used as his references. These include the *Shen Ying Jing (Divinely*

moxibustion) and was (in the process of) making a rigorous effort to convince and stimulate his subjects (in this art) when it so happened that from afar was presented not a rare, exotic plaything but a divine remedy book that can save the people and help the country. It unexpectedly arrived just (in time) to support His Majesty's prodigious virtue of benevolence toward his subjects and love for (all living) things. Its arrival was no accident.

Written by Han Ji-xi,
Bright Expositor of the Classics,
Loyally Devoted Crisis Settler,
Holder of the Pure and Righteous,
Merit-establishing Minister,
Great Man of Honor, West-Conquering Gentleman
21st (day), 11th month, 10th year of Cheng Hua[1]

---

[1] Cheng Hua (1465-1487 CE) was the name of the reign of Emperor Xian Zong of the Ming dynasty.

(Zhang Yun's) Preface to the
Shen Ying Jing

In the times of Tang and Yu[1], to brighten the establishment, no one except those who were strongly recommended as outstanding could become an official. In light of the establishment of Xi and Xuan[2], there would be no medicine without (such persons as) Shi Xiang[3], who specialized in the study of sound and whom even the sage honored as a teacher in music. As far as the study of medicine is concerned, I am an incompetent person. Therefore, I regret that I am inferior to old farmers.

---

[1]   Tang was the name of Yao, the first semi-legendary king in Chinese history, while Yu was Shun, who was the successor to Yao, the second king in Chinese history.

[2]   Xi refers to Fu Xi Shi, who, along with Huang Di and Shen Nong, is one of the three great culture heroes of the Chinese. It was Fu Xi who initiated the use of the *ba gua* or eight trigrams and was the first person to teach his people to fish and raise livestock and poultry. Xuan refers to Xuan Yuan Shi, *i.e.*, Huang Di or the Yellow Emperor. He defeated the belligerent tribe, the Chi You, and conquered the aggressive Yan Di (Flaming Emperor). Finally he was crowned by all the rival independent tribes as king. He is believed to be the forefather of the Han or Chinese nation.

[3]   Shi Xiang was a noted musician from whom Confucius once learned how to play musical instruments. One should note that Chinese medicine is closely associated with music in some respects. For instance, the complicated form of the word for herbs or medicinals, *yao*, is composed of the word for harmony surmounted by the grass radical. The word for harmony is itself composed of the picture of a drum on a wooden stand flanked by bells. Music is an entertainment for the heart to maintain peace and harmony.

However, from the time a human being is in possession of a body, because it is intoxicated by blood and qi, inundated by desire and lust, wrestling with cold and heat, and assaulted by all sorts of worries, scarcely a person is free from disease. Who except an exemplary person can remain safe? Accordingly, the sage devised and invented the remedy of stone needles and moxa. In the primitive ages, there were no medicinals and only the therapy of the stone needle and moxa was used. This saved the lives of people by the manipulation of the hands. This is a great medical *dao*. I am pleased with its ability to bring life back through the fingers alone without the bother of chewing and slicing associated with herbs. (Thus,) it should be said that (this method) is simple and convenient. For that reason, I appealed to physicians for books on this art, and, after a long time, I came into possession of (the works of) ten or more masters. Among these, only (Chen) Hong-gang, who met with and was imparted the art by the Immortal Xi Xin-qing, was distinct from physicians nowadays for his methods of supplementation and drainage, point measurement, wonderful rhymes, and wonderful finger manipulations. It is in these respects that he stands out above them. He had twenty-four pupils, among whom only Liu Jin grasped the secrets of his finger manipulation and, therefore, carried forward his art, not allowing it to relapse.

I have been contemplating that the Gan Jiang[4], though in the hands of a god, is not as good as an awl if it were used for mending a shoe. It is true that there are a wealth of efficacious medicinals, but they may not bring effect so rapidly as one single needle when used to thwart disease. Medicinals reach the disease by the strength of their qi and flavor. Therefore, they are

---

[4]   This is the name of a famous sword named after its maker, the smith Gan Jiang, who lived in the Spring and Autumn period (770-476 BCE). It is known as the most excellent sword that humans ever produced, and recent archaeological findings have proved this belief true.

slow in diffusing and disinhibiting the channels and connecting vessels. The needle takes the disease by means of puncturing and rubbing. Hence, it is quick in coursing and freeing the blood vessels. Moreover, there is the moxa cone. Ignited by the divine flint, it assists the true yang and dispels yin evils. Thus the original qi is replenished. (Having accomplished these ends,) what kind of disease may remain?

Suppose it is night or a person is travelling, a mild malady arises, and there are no medicinals available roundabout. Then only the art of the stone needle and moxa can cope with (such) an emergency. (Hence,) scholars who cherish the desire to treat life in the world should not be unfamiliar with (this art).

For that reason I have taken to and learned (this art). I instructed the scholar-physician, Liu Jin, to collate and recompile his master, (Chen) Hong-gang's ten volume *Guang Ai Shu (Book of Universal Love)*, but I chose to keep only those points most essential to practice to curtail the work to one volume and changed the title to the *Shen Ying Jing (The Divinely Responding Classic)*. It contains 548 disease patterns with 211 acupoints. In addition, 64 patterns with 145 acupoints based on Liu Jin's experience were elected and compiled as a separate book, titled the *Shen Ying Mi Yao (Secret Essentials of the Divinely Responding [Classic])*. With this endeavor, I wish to popularize the (loving) heart amidst the folks in order to live up to the compassion of universal love of (Chen) Hong-gang. This book has never been in existence in the world before. To bring it down, I ordered it put to press with this preface at the front.

Written by Zhang Yun
21st (day), 4th month, the year of Yi Si, Hong Xi[5]

---

5 Hong Xi was the name of the reign of the Emperor Ren Zong of the Ming dynasty who ruled the country for but one year. Yi Si was 1425 CE.

Table of Contents

Eight Point Moxa Method

I n the first month of winter, the ninth year of Cheng Hua, the year of Gui Si[1], Tonobukari, adjutant of Dono[2] Shimayama, Japan who sent the hermit Ryoshin over here, declared:

> Two hundred years ago my country boasted two distinguished physicians. One was Wasuke and the other was Niba. These two specialized in healing *yong* and *ju*, clove sores, furuncles, and large and small scrofulous lumps. They designed an eight point moxa method which is divinely efficacious.

The Eight Point Moxa Method

Two Points for the Head

(These treat) various kinds of sores breaking out on the head. Measure with a stalk of rice the circumference of the head at (the level of) the tips of the ears. [Start from the tip of the left ear, turn right, and, via the tip of the right ear, return to the starting point where the stalk should be broken off.] Put the stalk under the throat knot (*i.e.*, Adam's apple) with its ends at the back of the patient who is made to hold them with one hand, and then cut off the stalk. [Put the midpoint of the stalk under the Adam's apple and have its two ends meet at the nape of the neck. Have the ends downward and let the patient hold them in the hand, and then cut off the handgrip parts. This is

---

[1]   *I.e.*, 1474 CE.

[2]   This is a Japanese title of honor similar to the English (His) Highness.

similar to the method of one handsbreadth in the *Zhen Jing* {*Needle Classic*}³.] Mark the point on the spine where the stalk is cut. If the sores appear on the left side, moxa on the left, one half *cun* lateral to (the marked point on) the center of the spine. If the sores appear on the right, moxa on the right. If sores appear on both sides of the left and right (of the head), moxa on both sides.

Two Points for the Hand

(These treat) sores breaking out on the hand. Measure (with a stalk of rice) from the tip of the prominent shoulder bone [*i.e.*, Shoulder Bone, *Jian Yu*, LI 15] to the tip of the third (*i.e.*, middle) finger and cut it. Put the stalk under the throat knot with its two ends downward at the nape of the neck. Then proceed as in the case for the head.

Two Points for the Abdomen & Back

[From the Great Vertebra {*Da Zhui*, GV 14} down to the tip of the coccyx is the back, while from the Celestial Chimney {*Tian Tu*, CV 22} down to the edge of the pubic hair region is the abdomen. The regions under the armpits also belong to the abdominal-back precincts.] (These two points treat) sores breaking out on the back or abdomen. Measure (with a stalk of rice) the circumference above the breasts. [Start from above the left nipple and turn right to circle the body, returning to the starting point via the right nipple.] Put the stalk under the

---

³   *Zhen Jing* is another name for the *Ling Shu (Spiritual Pivot)*. However, the so-called method of one handsbreadth, which consists of measuring the breadth of the four fingers put together and equaling three body *cun*, was, in fact, invented by Sun Si-miao in his *Qian Jin Yao Fang (Prescriptions [Worth] a Thousand [Pieces of] Gold)* rather than by the Yellow Emperor in the *Ling Shu*.

throat knot with (its two ends) downward at the nape of the neck. Then proceed as in the case for the head.

Two Points for the Foot

(These treat) sores breaking out on the foot. Let (the patient) stand with the feet parallel and in contact. Measure (with a stalk of rice) the circumference from the tip of the left big toe to the tip of the right big toe. [Start from the tip of the left big toe, turn right {left?} along the edge of the {left} foot, pass the left and right heels, and return to the starting point via the tip of the right big toe.] Put the stalk under the throat knot with its ends downward at the nape of the neck. Then proceed as in the case for the head.

In moxaing these eight points, moxa till (the affected part) becomes painless if it is painful or moxa till (the affected part) becomes painful if it is painless. Or moxa with 500 or up to 800 cones. It is particularly good to moxa with a great many large cones. If *yong* and *ju* are (treated with) moxa at their initial stage, they will heal without festering. If they are (treated with) moxa when already festering, (new) flesh will be generated and their pain relieved. In addition, they will never relapse.

Shen Ying Ying
(Divinely Responding Classic)

Compiled by Elder-born[1] (Chen) Hong-gang
(a.k.a.) Chen Hui (Chen Shan-tong)

Collated and Recompiled by
Official Physician Liu Jin (Liu Yong-huai)

Elder-born (Chen) Hong-gang said, "When great carpenters teach people, they present them with compasses and squares but (nevertheless, they) are unable to make them skillful." He was engaged in needling for forty years, during which time, whenever he occasionally met with someone who did not despise (this art), he would try to elucidate it, endeavoring to make them see the light yet always fearing that the instructed did not appreciate it fully.

At first he wrote a book of twelve volumes, the *Guang Ai Shu (The Book of Universal Love)*. Illustrating it with poems and rhymes, he (initially) thought the book left out little to be desired. However, he became concerned that the work was so vast in scope and touched such a wide (variety of topics) that the reader might become bored of reading and tired of its study

---

[1] Elder-born is the literal translation of the Chinese *xian sheng*. In modern usage, this is usually translated as Mister. However, Elder-born conveys the Confucian concern for filial piety this term implies and the general Chinese reverence for age. In addition, Mister would be anachronistic in translating a classic from this period.

due to its complexity. Therefore, they might not work their way to eventual success.

Nonetheless, the *dao* is handed down in words and books teach (through the medium of) words. Because of this, (I) picked out what must be learned by heart and compiled it as the *Guang Ai Shu Kuo (A Summarization of the Book of Universal Love)*. Compact as it is, (I) still had the misgiving that readers might not comprehend the essential fundamentals. Thus they may feel sorrow as if peeping through a wall. For that reason, barely 119 points were chosen, illustrated by poems and pictures. Thus, we collected the most essential points for the treatment of disease to present to learners in a one volume book as a set of squares and compasses. Since this should be said to be the most concise of concise works, one is expected to study it closely and familiarize (themselves) with it (thoroughly). If one wants to be a divine, holy, skillful, or clever practitioner with a penetrating eye, one is required (even) more.

The key lies in a thorough understanding (of the text) and the ability to act in accordance with specific conditions. When one meets with a situation difficult to grasp through a (mere) explanation in words, one should leave it open till one acquires true knowledge. When one builds up enough experience, one will eventually (understand. Therefore,) this (book) has been specially (*i.e.,* only) written to show learners the right direction to go.

Supplementing & Draining Manipulation

Your servant, (Liu) Jin, commented: Acupuncture and moxibustion's ability to affect the feat of thwarting disease entirely depends on the *shou fa* or manual manipulation. (Granted,) unless the right position of the point is located, this feat will not be accomplished in any case. (However,) suppose the right position of the point is located but supplementation and drainage are carried out in a wrong way, the effort will be nonetheless in vain.

Elder-born (Chen) Hong-gang said: According to the popularly known supplementing and draining methods, supplementation is to turn the (manipulating) thumb outward, while drainage is to turn it inward. This is a gross fallacy. What the vulgar practitioners call drainage is actually a supplementing needling method. What they call supplementation is actually a draining needling method. One should be aware that, in terms of supplementing and draining methods, for the left side of the body there is one method and for the right there is another. Treating in the direction of the flow of qi and blood is an irrational approach. What to treat?

He also said that it is stated in the *Su Wen (Simple Questions)* that needling holds back moxibustion and moxibustion holds back needling. The charlatan adds moxibustion to needling and adds needling to moxibustion. There have been some among the later generations who did not have an idea of the teachings of the Yellow Emperor and Qi Bo and crowned needling with moxibustion and moxibustion with needling. It should be understood that, when in their (*i.e.,* the Yellow Emperor and Qi Bo's) work, a certain point is described in a (certain) location and admits of being needled to a certain number of *fen* deep or moxaed with a certain number of cones, this means that, if needling, such a depth may be reached and, if moxaing, so many cones may be used. This does not imply that the point should be needled after being moxaed or moxaed after being needled.

Nowadays, in administering moxibustion, practitioners invariably moxa three cones first, then needle, and finally repeat moxaing with several (more) cones. This method is called penetrating fire. Such an approach to moxibustion reveals an ignorance of the implications in the book (*i.e.,* the *Su Wen*) and a lack of awareness of the purport of the Yellow Emperor and Qi Bo. This is deeply deplorable. As pointed out in the *Zhuang*[1], "Those who are stupid (usually) insist on their own way." There are indeed such persons. In the past, Elder-born (Chen) Hong-gang often explained that only (those points) on the abdomen allow moxaing with a number of cones immediately following in the wake of needling. This is in order to fortify those points. This is alright (for points on the abdomen), but it is forbidden for points on other parts of the body. One cannot apply a (single) example everywhere, and one should be conscious of this medical approach to (the practice of) discretion.

Illustration of the Technique of Drainage

Your servant (Liu) Jin commented: According to Elder-born Hong-gang's instructions, after exactly locating a point, one should press it with the left thumb and place the needle on it with the right hand. Bid the patient to let out a cough and, with the coughing, insert the needle to the right depth. Pause for a while after all the needles are inserted into the (required)

---

[1] *I.e., Commentaries (on the Classic of Change)*

points. Holding one between the right thumb and forefinger, gently rock it to make it advance and retreat while turning it with the hand as if trembling. This is known as hastening the qi. After manipulating this way 5-6 times, when the qi around the needle is felt to tighten, perform the draining method: If the left side is needled, hold the needle between the right thumb and forefinger, moving the thumb forward and the forefinger backward to lift the needle a bit while turning it toward the left.

If more than one needle is inserted, all of them should be so manipulated in turn. Then, still holding an (inserted) needle between the right thumb and forefinger, roll the forefinger thrice. This is known as flying (or flapping). Proceed by still gently raising the needle while turning it toward the left until it has retreated about one half *fen*. This is called triple flapping with one single retreat. Perform this maneuver 5-6 times till the needle feels heavy and tight. By now, the qi is arriving to an extreme extent. Then continue to lift the needle a bit while giving it one or two turns to the left.

If the right side is needled, hold the needle between the left thumb and forefinger, moving the thumb forward and the forefinger backward, and then roll the needle thrice as instructed above. Lifting the needle a bit while turning it toward the right is the draining method for needling the right side.

When one is about to extract the needle, one should bid the patient to let out a cough and, with the coughing, withdraw it. This is the so-called draining method.

Illustration of the Technique of Supplementation

Your servant (Liu) Jin comments: Once Elder-born Hong-gang taught that disease in people is invariably due to the convergence of evil qi. (Therefore,) even in the case of a thin, emaciated patient, one should not exclusively use the supplementing

9

method. The classic (*i.e.*, the *Nei Jing [Inner Classic]*) says, "Wherever evil converges, the qi is invariably vacuous." Suppose, (however,) there is the disorder of red eyes. Since this is evidently caused by evil heat, it is permissible to exclusively perform the draining method. As to other kinds of illness (consisting of mixed vacuity and repletion), it is appropriate only to carry out balanced supplementation and drainage. (In this case,) it is proper that drainage take precedence over supplementation. (This is) called the method of draining evils before supplementing the true qi. This is the secret of his success that was never imparted (to anyone else).

If one is found ill, manipulate the needle as instructed above to hasten and secure the qi. After drainage is completed, perform the supplementing method. Bid the patient to inhale a mouthful of air and, with the inhalation, turn the needle. If the left side is needled, turn the needle to the right, holding the needle between the right thumb and forefinger. (In this case,) the forefinger moves forward and the thumb backward. Turn the needle 1-2 *fen* deeper to cause the true qi to penetrate into the division (*i.e.*, depth) of the muscle and flesh.

If the right side is needled, turn the needle to the left, holding the needle between the left thumb and forefinger. (In this case,) move the forefinger forward and the thumb backward. Continue to push the needle 1-2 *fen* deeper by turning. If more than one point is needled, perform this maneuver on all the points. After completion, pause for a short while. Then flick the end of the needle with a finger three times. This procedure should be done thrice. Then, still holding the needle between the left thumb and forefinger, roll the thumb three times. This is called flapping and lets the needle go 1-2 *fen* deeper. (During this process,) the needle is turned toward the left. This is called one advance with three flaps. Perform this maneuver as instructed 5-6 times till the needle feels heavy and tight or till the qi around the needle becomes hot.

10

By now the qi is abundant. Bid the patient to inhale a mouthful of air. While inhaling, extract the needle and then press the point with the hand (*i.e.*, a finger) promptly. This is known as the supplementing method.

The Fourfold Flower-like
Point Moxaing Method[1]

The first two points:

First have the patient stand erect. Obtain a thread which is waxed to prevent it from stretching and contracting. Fix one end to the tip of the big toe, the left for men and the right for women. Turn the thread around the heel through the sole and, passing the calf, draw it upward to the midpoint of the large transverse crease at the popliteal fossa where the thread is cut off. Bid the patient to loosen and part (his or her) hair with the dividing line made visible from the fontanel to the back of the head. Then have the patient sit straight. Press one end of the thread to the tip of the patient's nose, drawing the thread upward, running it to the back of the head along the dividing line of the hair, and then running it downward, (the thread being) in contact with the skin all the way. Mark with ink the point where the thread ends on the central line of the spine. In the case of a woman with bound feet[2], which is a practice against the law of natural growth, if the feet were taken as (part of) the measure, the length (of the thread) will be inadequate. In that case, locate the Shoulder Bone Point (*Jian Yu*, LI 15), press one end of the thread on it, make the patient stretch her hand,

---

[1]   Modern acupuncturists call the points Diaphragm Shu (*Ge Shu*, Bl 17) and Gallbladder Shu (*Dan Shu*, Bl 19) the Four Flowers Points. This method should not be confused with that group of points.

[2]   In old China, girls' feet were tightly bound from childhood in order to stunt their growth.

and draw the thread down to the tip of the middle finger where the thread is cut for (the measurement of the four flowers) point. This is also applicable in males.

(Next,) bid the patient shut their mouth. Press one end of a short waxed thread on the left corner of the mouth, draw the thread up to the root of the nose, and then turn it down slantwise to the right corner of the mouth, making the thread into a triangle. Cut it off at the right corner of the mouth. Straighten the thread and then bend it to find its midpoint which is (then) marked with ink. Overlay the ink-marked midpoint of the thread on the ink-marked point on the spine, fixing the two ends of the thread (which is set crosswise). Be careful not to let the (operating) hands slip higher or lower. Circle the points in ink where the two ends of the thread are. These are two desired points. The above is the first two-point marking.

The next two points:

Bid the patient to sit straight with their arms a little bent. Put a waxed thread around the (patient's) neck, hanging it on the large vertebra (C7) with its two ends meeting at the tip of the turtledove's bone (*i.e.*, the xiphoid process). In persons without a xiphoid process, one *cun* from the branched bone (*i.e.*, the 7th costosternal articulation) in the chest can be taken as the turtledove's bone. There, cut off the ends. Then turn round the thread to have its ends at the back. Pressing (its midpoint) on the Adam's apple, pass the thread by either side of the neck and align it with the spine. Mark in ink the point where the ends are. Bid the patient to shut their mouth. Put a short waxed thread through the mouth to measure its width. Cut it at the two corners of the mouth. As instructed above, bend the thread to have its midpoint and put the point on the ink-marked point on the spine. Measure crosswise as instructed above. Circle in

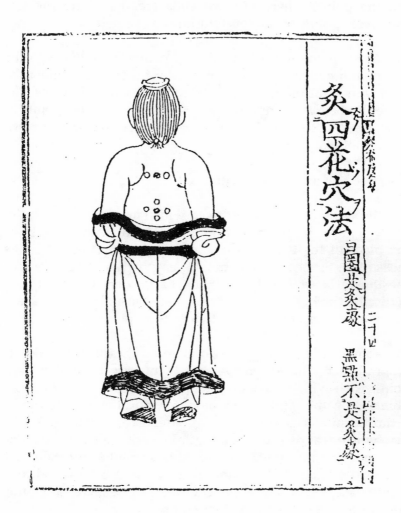

Illustration Showing the Location
of the Fourfold Flower-like Points

ink the points where the two ends are. These are the two transverse points of the fourfold flower-like points.

The above is the second marking of points. Together with the first marking, there are four points. Moxa them simultaneously, each with 7 to 2 times 7 cones, 120 cones, or even 150 cones. The more the better. Do not moxa the next two (sets of) points as instructed (below) until moxa sores break out (on the first two sets of points).

The further next two points:

Use the second time's short thread which measured the mouth. Press its midpoint on the ink-marked point on the spine. This is the place of the two ends of the thread in the second time's measuring. Set the thread straight lengthwise. Make sure that the thread is set exactly upright. The two ends (should) rest vertically. Circle in ink the points where the ends are. These are the two vertical points of the four flowers points.

The above is the third marking of points. (These three markings are) called the fourfold flower-like points. Moxa the (last) two points each with 100 cones. These three markings produce six points altogether. Choose fire days[3] for moxaing. In addition, it is most desirable that the Folium Artemisiae Argyii (*Ai Ye*) be that which was picked up on the 3rd day of the 3rd month. For 100 days after moxaing, one should be careful about their diet and sexual affairs. (They should) repose in a calm mood in a quiet place. Should the patient not feel relieved a month afterwards, moxa again the first points.

---

[3]   *Bing* (S3) and *ding* (S4) days in the 10 day cycle correspond to the fire phase and are thus so-called fire days.

The Category of Various Winds

F or paralysis of the left or right legs: Pool at the Bend (*Qu Chi*, LI 11), Yang Ravine (*Yang Xi*, LI 5), Union Valley (*He Gu*, LI 4), Central Flow (*Zhong Zhu*, Ki 15), (Leg) Three *Li* (*San Li*, St 36), Yang Assistance (*Yang Fu*, GB 38), and Kunlun (Mountain, *Kun Lun*, Bl 60)

For inability to bend the elbow: Wrist Bone (*Wan Gu*, SI 4)

For feet without fatty sheen (*i.e.*, for dry, lusterless feet): Upper Ridge (*Shang Lian*, St 37)

For hemilateral wind: Broken Sequence (*Lie Que*, Lu 7) and Surging Yang (*Chong Yang*, St 42)

For arch-backed rigidity with limb hypertonicity: Liver *Shu* (*Gan Shu*, Bl 18)

For spasm of the elbow in wind stroke: Inner Pass (*Nei Guan*, Per 6)

For up-turned eyes: Silk Bamboo Hole (*Si Zhu Kong*, TH 23)

For foaming at the mouth: Silk Bamboo Hole (*Si Zhu Kong*, TH 23) and Hundred Convergences (*Bai Hui*, GV 20)

For inability to recognize people: Water Trough (*Shui Gou*, GV 26), (Head) Overlooking Tears (*Lin Qi*, GB 15), and Union Valley (*He Gu*, LI 4)

For arch-backed rigidity: Mute's Gate (*Ya Men*, CV 15) and Wind Mansion (*Feng Fu*, GV 16)

For wind *bi*[1]: Celestial Well (*Tian Jing*, TH 10), Cubit Marsh, (*Chi Ze*, Lu 5), Lesser Sea (*Shao Hai*, Ht 3), Bend Middle (*Wei Zhong*, Bl 40), and Yang Assistance (*Yang Fu*, GB 38)

For fright epilepsy: Cubit Marsh (*Chi Ze*, Lu 5) [1 cone], Lesser Surge (*Shao Chong*, Ht 9), Before the Vertex (*Qian Ding*, GV 21), and Bundle Bone (*Shu Gu*, Bl 65)

For wind epilepsy[2]: Spirit Court (*Shen Ting*, GV 24), Hundred Convergences (*Bai Hui*, GV 20), Before the Vertex (*Qian Ding*, GV 21), Gushing Spring (*Yong Quan*, Ki 1), Silk Bamboo Hole (*Si Zhu Kong*, TH 23), Spirit Gate (*Shen Que*, CV 8) [1 cone],and Turtle-dove Tail (*Jiu Wei*, CV 15) [3 cones]

For wind taxation[3]: Spring at the Bend (*Qu Quan*, Liv 8) and Bladder *Shu* (*Pang Guang Shu*, Bl 28) [7 cones]

---

[1] This is also called migratory *bi*. The main symptom of migratory *bi* is aching in the limbs which moves about and is not fixed.

[2] Wind epilepsy is a particular type of epilepsy. Its distinctive manifestations include susceptibility to fright, and, during attacks, dilated pupils, tremors of the extremities, crying in one's sleep, and body heat besides other symptoms common to epilepsy in general. It is caused by heart qi vacuity accompanied by accumulated heat and invasion of wind.

[3] Wind taxation is a kind of vacuity detriment resulting from long consumption of qi and blood. At its beginning, wind cold intrudes into the body, resulting in painful *bi* and numbness. If this is not treated properly, evils enter the bowels and further affect the viscera, consuming qi and blood.

For wind pouring[4]: Hundred Convergences (*Bai Hui*, GV 20) [2 cones], Liver *Shu* (*Gan Shu*, Bl 18) [3 cones], Spleen *Shu* (*Pi Shu*, Bl 20) [3 cones], Kidney *Shu* (*Shen Shu*, Bl 23) [the same number of cones as years of age], and Bladder *Shu* (*Pang Guang Shu*, Bl 28)

For wind dizziness[5]: (Head) Overlooking Tears (*Lin Qi*, GB 15), Yang Valley (*Yang Gu*, SI 5), Wrist Bone (*Wan Gu*, SI 4), and Extending Vessel (*Shen Mai*, Bl 62)

For pain in wind stroke: (Head) Overlooking Tears (*Lin Qi*, GB 15), Hundred Convergences (*Bai Hui*, GV 20), Shoulder Well (*Jian Jing*, GB 21), Shoulder Bone (*Jian Yu*, LI 15), Pool at the Bend (*Qu Chi*, LI 11), Celestial Well (*Tian Jing*, TH 10), Intermediary Courier (*Jian Shi*, Per 5), Inner Pass (*Nei Guan*, Per 6), Union Valley (*He Gu*, LI 4), Wind Market (*Feng Shi*, GB 31), (Leg) Three Li (*San Li*, St 36), Ravine Divide (*Jie Xi*, St 41), Kunlun (Mountain, *Kun Lun*, Bl 60), and Shining Sea (*Zhao Hai*, Ki 6)

For loss of voice and muteness: Branch Ditch (*Zhi Gou*, TH 6), Recover Flow (*Fu Liu*, Ki 7), Intermediary Courier (*Jian Shi*, Per 5), Union Valley (*He Gu*, LI 4), Fish Border (*Yu Ji*, Lu 10), Spirit Pathway (*Ling Dao*, Ht 4), Yin Valley (*Yin Gu*, Ki 10), Blazing Valley (*Ran Gu*, Ki 2), and Valley Passage (*Tong Gong*, Bl 66)

For clenched jaw and shut mouth: Jawbone (*Jia Che*, St 6), Sauce Receptacle (*Cheng Jiang*, CV 24), and Union Valley (*He Gu*, LI 4)

---

4   Wind pouring refers to evil qi moving up and down and around the body with the defensive and constructive qi. This causes a migratory, aching pain in the skin.

5   Wind dizziness is a type of dizziness of the head with flowery vision and counterflow which, over time, may develop into epilepsy. It is due to qi and blood vacuity and wind evils intruding into the brain.

For the wind epilepsy disease of lying down unconscious on the ground in every attack: Moxa Wind Pool (*Feng Chi*, GB 20) and Hundred Convergences (*Bai Hui*, GV 20).

The Yellow Emperor asked Qi Bo:

How should one moxa when a person is taken with wind stroke with hemiplegia?

Qi Bo answered:

If occasional sudden aching and cheek *bi* arise two or 3-5 months before contraction of wind stroke and these do not resolve till long after, these are signs of forthcoming wind stroke. It is (therefore) necessary to promptly moxa (Leg) Three *Li* (*San Li*, St 36) and Severed Bone (*Jue Gu*, GB 39), four points altogether, each with 3 cones. (Then) spray and wash the moxa sores with a decoction of Herba Menthae (*Bo He*) and Folium Polygoni Multiflori (*Tao Liu Ye*) to drive the wind qi from out of the sore openings.

If the moxa sores heal in spring, moxa (these points) again in autumn. If the sores heal in autumn, moxa (these points) again in spring. It is desirable to keep moxa sores on the two legs all the time. If one does not believe in this method, is undisciplined in food and drink, or overindulges in wine and sex, one may be suddenly struck by this kind of wind with sluggish or difficult speech and hemiplegia. (In this case,) it is appropriate to moxa the following seven points each with 3 cones:

If the wind is located on the right side, moxa the left (points). If it is on the left, moxa the right. The first is Hundred Convergences (*Bai Hui*, GV 20). The second is the hairlines anterior to the ears (*i.e.*, moxa both hairlines in front of the ears). The third is Shoulder Well (*Jian Jing*, GB 21). The fourth is Wind Market (*Feng Shi*, GB 31). The fifth is (Leg) Three *Li* (*San Li*, St 36). The sixth is Severed Bone (*Jue Gu*, GB 39). The seventh is Pool at the Bend (*Qu Chi*, LI 11).

The above seven points are miraculously effective for many (diseases). Moxa as instructed and there will not be a single failure out of ten thousand cases.

The Yellow Emperor's moxaing method to treat wind stroke with upturned eyes and loss of speech: Moxa at the 3rd (2nd in a variant version; tr.) and 5th (thoracic) vertebrae, 7 cones apiece. These should be as big as half a date seed.

The Category of Cold Damage

For body heat and headache: Bamboo Gathering (*Zan Zhu*, Bl 2), Great Mound (*Da Ling*, Per 7), Spirit Gate (*Shen Men*, Ht 7), Union Valley (*He Gu*, LI 4), Fish Border (*Yu Ji*, Lu 10), Central Islet (*Zhong Zhu*, TH 3), Humor Gate (*Ye Men*, TH 2), Lesser Marsh (*Shao Ze*, SI 1), Bend Middle (*Wei Zhong*, Bl 40), and Supreme White (*Tai Bai*, Sp 3)

For aversion to cold as after a soaking and shuddering and chattering with cold: Fish Border (*Yu Ji*, Lu 10)

For body heat (*i.e.*, generalized fever): Sunken Valley (*Xian Gu*, St 43), Small Lu (*Lu Xi*, Ki 3) [do not extract the needle till the cold in the feet has reached the knees], (Leg) Three *Li* (*San Li*, St 36), Recover Flow (*Fu Liu*, Ki 7), Pinched Ravine (*Xia Xi*, GB 43), Offspring of the Noble (*Gong Sun*, Sp 4)[1], Supreme White (*Tai Bai*, Sp 3), Bend Middle (*Wei Zhong*, Bl 40), and Gushing Spring (*Yong Quan*, Ki 1)

For (alternating) cold and heat: Wind Pool (*Feng Chi*, GB 20), Lesser Sea (*Shao Hai*, Ht 3), Fish Border (*Yu Ji*, Lu 10), Lesser Surge (*Shao Chong*, Ht 9), Union Valley (*He Gu*, LI 4), Recover Flow (*Fu Liu*, Ki 7), (Head) Overlooking Tears (*Lin Qi*, GB 15), and Supreme White (*Tai Bai*, Sp 3)

---

[1] According to Nigel Wiseman *et al.*'s terminology, this point's name should be translated as Yellow Emperor. This is one of the few point name translations coined by them that the translator cannot bring himself to use. See the discussion in the Translator's Preface.

For cold damage with sweat refusing to exude: Wind Pool (*Feng Chi*, GB 20), Fish Border (*Yu Ji*, Lu 10), and Channel Ditch (*Jing Gu*, Lu 8) [drain each] and Second Space (*Er Jian*, LI 2)

For channel passage delay[2]: Cycle Gate (*Qi Men*, Liv 14)

For persistent remaining heat: Pool at the Bend (*Qu Chi*, LI 11), (Arm) Three *Li* (*San Li*, LI 10), and Union Valley (*He Gu*, LI 4)

For abdominal distention: (Leg) Three *Li* (*San Li*, St 36) and Inner Court (*Nei Ting*, St 44)

For yin pattern cold damage[3]: Moxa Spirit Gate (*Shen Que*, CV 8) [200-300 cones].

For great heat: Pool at the Bend (*Qu Chi*, LI 11), (Arm) Three *Li* (*San Li*, LI 10), and Recover Flow (*Fu Liu*, Ki 7)

For retching and vomiting: Hundred Convergences (*Bai Hui*, GV 20), Marsh at the Bend (*Qu Ze*, Per 3), Intermediary Courier (*Jian Shi*, Per 5), Palace of Toil (*Lao Gong*, Per 8), and Shang Hill (*Shang Qiu*, Sp 5)

For cold in the abdomen with heat qi (in the exterior): Lesser Surge (*Shao Chong*, Ht 9), Shang Hill (*Shang Qiu*, Sp 5), Supreme

---

2 If, after the *tai yang* channel pattern of cold damage should have resolved itself, a desire to vomit, chest pain, slight vexation, abdominal fullness, and diarrhea appear, this is called channel passage delay. This may be due to either an unusual progression of the *tai yang* pattern or, as in most cases, is the result of inappropriate administration of precipitating or ejecting (*i.e.*, promoting vomiting) therapies.

3 If a cold damage passes over the yang (*tai yang*, *yang ming*, and *shao yang*) phases and straight away hit the yin phase, giving a yin pattern of manifestations, this is called yin pattern cold damage.

Surge (*Tai Chong*, Liv 3), Moving Between (*Xing Jian*, Liv 2), Three Yin Intersection (*San Yin Jiao*, Sp 6), Hidden White (*Yin Bai*, Sp 1), and Yin Mound Spring (*Yin Ling Quan*, Sp 9) [3 cones]

For mania: Hundred Taxations (*Bai Lao*, GV 14), Intermediary Courier (*Jian Shi*, Per 5), Union Valley (*He Gu*, LI 4), and Recover Flow (*Fu Liu*, Ki 7) [all moxaed]

For unconsciousness of human affairs: Central Islet (*Zhong Zhu*, TH 3), (Leg) Three *Li* (*San Li*, St 36), and Great Pile (*Da Dun*, Liv 1)

For constipation: Shining Sea (*Zhao Hai*, Ki 6) and Screen Gate (*Zhang Men*, Liv 13)

For urinary stoppage: Yin Valley (*Yin Gu*, Ki 10) and Yin Mound Spring (*Yin Ling Quan*, Sp 9)

The Category of Phlegm, Dyspnea & Coughing

F or coughing: Broken Sequence (*Lie Que*, Lu 7), Channel Ditch (*Jing Qu*, Lu 8), Cubit Marsh (*Chi Ze*, Lu 5), Fish Border (*Yu Ji*, Lu 10), Lesser Marsh (*Shao Ze*, SI 1), Front Valley (*Qian Gu*, SI 2), (Leg) Three *Li* (*San Li*, St 36), Ravine Divide (*Jie Xi*, St 41), Kunlun (Mountain, *Kun Lun*, Bl 60), Lung *Shu* (*Fei Shu*, Bl 13) [100 cones], and Chest Center (*Dan Zhong*, CV 17) [7 cones]

For coughing with swelling[1]: Great Abyss (*Tai Yuan*, Lu 9)

For dragging costal pain (on coughing): Liver *Shu* (*Gan Shu*, Bl 18)

For dragging pain in the sacrum and coccyx (in coughing): Fish Border (*Yu Ji*, Lu 10)

For coughing with blood: Broken Sequence (*Lie Que*, Lu 7), (Leg) Three *Li* (*San Li*, St 36), Lung *Shu* (*Fei Shu*, Bl 13), Hundred Taxations (*Bai Lao*, M-HN-30), Breast Root (*Ru Gen*, St 18), Wind Gate (*Feng Men*, Bl 12), and Liver *Shu* (*Gan Shu*, Bl 18)

For spitting of blood with internal detriment: Fish Border (*Yu Ji*, Lu 10) [drain], Cubit Marsh (*Chi Ze*, Lu 5) [supplement], Intermediary Courier (*Jian Shi*, Per 5), Spirit Gate (*Shen Men*, Ht 7), Great Abyss (*Tai Yuan*, Lu 9), Palace of Toil (*Lao Gong*, Per 8),

---

[1] Because of the ambiguity of this term in Chinese, it may also plausibly be rendered by (massive) drinking instead of swelling.

27

Spring at the Bend (*Qu Quan*, Liv 8), Great Ravine (*Tai Xi*, Ki 3), Blazing Valley (*Ran Gu*, Ki 2), Supreme Surge (*Tai Chong*, Liv 3), Lung *Shu* (*Fei Shu*, Bl 13) [100 cones], Liver *Shu* (*Gan Shu*, Bl 18) [3 cones], and Spleen *Shu* (*Pi Shu*, Bl 20) [2 cones]

For spitting of blood with shivering from cold: Great Ravine (*Tai Xi*, Ki 3), (Leg) Three *Li* (*San Li*, St 36), Broken Sequence (*Lie Que*, Lu 7), and Great Abyss (*Tai Yuan*, Lu 9)

For retching of blood: Marsh at the Bend (*Qu Ze*, Per 3), Spirit Gate (*Shen Men*, Ht 7), and Fish Border (*Yu Ji*, Lu 10)

For retching of pus: Chest Center (*Dan Zhong*, CV 17)

For spitting of turbidity: Cubit Marsh (*Chi Ze*, Lu 5), Intermediary Courier (*Jian Shi*, Per 5), Broken Sequence (*Lie Que*, Lu 7), and Lesser Shang (*Shao Shang*, Lu 11)

For retching and inability to transform food: Supreme White (*Tai Bai*, Sp 3)

For retching and vomiting: Marsh at the Bend (*Qu Ze*, Per 3), Connecting the Interior (*Tong Li*, Ht 5), Palace of Toil (*Lao Gong*, Per 8), Yang Mound (Spring) (*Yang Ling*, GB 34), Great Ravine (*Tai Xi*, Ki 3), Shining Sea (*Zhao Hai*, Ki 6), Supreme Surge (*Tai Chong*, Liv 3), Great Metropolis (*Da Du*, Sp 2), Hidden White (*Yin Bai*, Sp 1), Open Valley (*Tong Gu*, Ki 20), Stomach *Shu* (*Wei Shu*, Bl 21), and Lung *Shu* (*Fei Shu*, Bl 13)

For counterflow retching[2]: Great Mound (*Da Ling*, Per 7)

---

[2] This simply refers to retching. Counterflow indicates the cause of the disorder, *i.e.*, the stomach failing to downbear qi. This qi then goes upward instead, bringing with it the contents of the stomach and producing a sound.

For retching and vomiting: Great Abyss (*Tai Yuan*, Lu 9)

For dyspnea, retching, and yawning and stretching: Channel Ditch (*Jing Gu*, Lu 8)

For (qi) ascension dyspnea: Marsh at the Bend (*Qu Ze*, Per 3), Great Mound (*Da Ling*, Per 7), Spirit Gate (*Shen Men*, Ht 7), Fish Border (*Yu Ji*, Lu 10), Third Space (*San Jian*, LI 3), Shang Yang (*Shang Yang*, LI 1), Ravine Divide (*Jie Xi*, St 41), Kunlun (Mountain, *Kun Lun*, Bl 60), Chest Center (*Dan Zhong*, CV 17), and Lung *Shu* (*Fei Shu*, Bl 13)

For frequent yawning with dyspnea: Great Abyss (*Tai Yuan*, Lu 9)

For coughing and dyspnea and blocked food[3]: Diaphragm *Shu* (*Ge Shu*, Bl 17)

For dyspnea and fullness: Third Space (*San Jian*, LI 3) and Shang Yang (*Shang Yang*, LI 1)

For lung inflating distention with qi surging and heat and pain all over the flanks: Yin Metropolis (*Yin Du*, Ki 19) [moxa], Great Abyss (*Tai Yuan*, Lu 9), and Lung *Shu* (*Fei Shu*, Bl 13)

For dyspneic breathing with inability to move about: Central Venter (*Zhong Wan*, CV 12), Cycle Gate (*Qi Men*, Liv 14), and Upper Ridge (*Shang Lian*, St 39)

---

[3] This is a mild kind of esophageal constriction which manifests with reflux of food upon ingestion.

For various kinds of vacuity and detriment, the five types of taxation[4], the seven types of damage[5], and essence loss taxation pattern[6]: Shoulder Well (*Jian Jing*, GB 21), Great Vertebra (*Da Zhui*, GV 14), *Gao Huang* (*Gao Huang*, Bl 43), Spleen *Shu* (*Pi Shu*, Bl 20), Stomach *Shu* (*Wei Shu*, Bl 21), Lung *Shu* (*Fei Shu*, Bl 13), Lower Venter (*Xia Wan*, CV 10), and (Leg) Three *Li* (*San Li*, St 36)

For cadaverine transmission, steaming bone, and lung atony[7]: *Gao Huang* (*Gao Huang*, Bl 43), Lung *Shu* (*Fei Shu*, Bl 13), and Fourfold Flower-like Points (*Si Hua Xue, i.e.,* Diaphragm *Shu* [*Ge Shu*, Bl 17], and Liver *Shu* [*Gan Shu*, Bl 18])

---

[4] *I.e.,* heart, liver, spleen, lung, and kidney taxation. Heart taxation is manifested by insomnia, sleep fraught with dreams, and other neurotic disorders. Liver taxation, which is caused by emotional disturbance, is manifested by dizziness, chest distention, anxiety, delirium, illusion, insomnia, and some other mental disorders. Spleen taxation is a disease of low food intake, untransformed food in stools, diarrhea, abdominal distention, and other digestive disorders. Lung taxation can refer either to consumptive disease or damage done to the lungs. It is manifested by cough, chest oppression and fullness, and distressed rapid dyspneic breathing. Kidney taxation, a problem caused by excessive food intake and overindulging in sex, is manifested by loss of essence with dreams, dizziness, ringing in the ears, vexing heat in the palms of the hands and soles of the feet, weakness and pain of the low back and knees, etc.

[5] The seven damages refer to the spleen being damaged by overeating, the liver being damaged by great anger and resultant qi counterflow, the kidneys being damaged by lifting heavy weights and sitting on the damp ground, the lungs being damaged by cold form and drinking cold substances, and the heart being damaged by worry and anxiety.

[6] This is a vacuity taxation pattern with essence loss, *i.e.,* spermatorrhea, as its main manifestation.

[7] Cadaverine transmission refers to an epidemic, infectious disease.

For dry retching: Intermediary Courier (*Jian Shi*, Per 5) [30 cones], Gallbladder *Shu* (*Dan Shu*, Bl 19), Valley Passage (*Tong Gu*, Bl 66), and Hidden White (*Yin Bai*, Sp 1). (In addition,) moxa 1.5 *cun* under the nipples.

For belching: Spirit Gate (*Shen Men*, Ht 7), Great Abyss (*Tai Yuan*, Lu 9), Lesser Shang (*Shao Shang*, Lu 11), Palace of Toil (*Lao Gong*, Per 8), Great Ravine (*Tai Xi*, Ki 3), Sunken Valley (*Xian Gu*, St 43), Supreme White (*Tai Bai*, Sp 3), and Great Pile (*Da Dun*, Liv 1)

For (copious) phlegm and drooling: Yin Valley (*Yin Gu*, Ki 10), Blazing Valley (*Ran Gu*, Ki 2), and Recover Flow (*Fu Liu*, Ki 7)

For bound accumulation and retained rheum: Diaphragm *Shu* (*Ge Shu*, Bl 17) [5 cones] and Open Valley (*Tong Gu*, Ki 20) [moxa]

The Category of Various Accumulations & Gatherings

F or qi lumps, cold qi, and all kinds of qi illness: Sea of Qi (*Qi Hai*, CV 6)

For heart qi pain radiating to the flanks: Hundred Convergences (*Bai Hui*, GV 20), Upper Venter (*Shang Wan*, CV 13), Branch Ditch (*Zhi Gou*, TH 6), Great Mound (*Da Ling*, Per 7), and (Arm) Three *Li* (*San Li*, LI 10)[1]

For bound qi ascension dyspnea and deep-lying beam qi[2]: Central Venter (*Zhong Wan*, CV 12)

For cup-like (glomus fullness) under the heart: Central Venter (*Zhong Wan*, CV 12) and Hundred Convergences (*Bai Hui*, GV 20)

For accumulated qi in the lateral costal regions: Cycle Gate (*Qi Men*, Liv 14)

---

[1]   One should note that Leg Three *Li* (*Zu San Li*, St 36) is also effective for this problem.

[2]   In premodern Chinese medical texts, qi, as it is here, is often no more than a synonym for illness or disease. Deep-lying beam is another name for heart *ji* or cardiac accumulation. This is manifested by fullness and hardness of the upper abdomen with seemingly roots on all sides. One should note that deep-lying beam may also occur in the lower abdomen as well.

For running piglet qi[3]: Screen Gate (*Zhang Men*, Liv 13), Cycle Gate (*Qi Men*, Liv 14), Central Venter (*Zhong Wan*, CV 12), Great Tower Gate (*Ju Que*, CV 14), and Sea of Qi (*Qi Hai*, CV 6) [100 cones]

For qi counterflow: Cubit Marsh (*Chi Ze*, Lu 5), Shang Hill (*Shang Qiu*, Sp 5), Supreme White (*Tai Bai*, Sp 3), and Three Yin Intersection (*San Yin Jiao*, Sp 6)

For counterflow dyspnea: Spirit Gate (*Shen Men*, Ht 7), Yin Mound (Spring) (*Yin Ling*, Sp 9), Kunlun (Mountain, *Kun Lun*, Bl 60), and Foot Overlooking Tears (*Zu Lin Qi*, GB 41)

For (qi) ascension counterflow belching: Great Abyss (*Tai Yuan*, Lu 9) and Spirit Gate (*Shen Men*, Ht 7)

For counterflow coughing: Branch Ditch (*Zhi Gou*, TH 6), Front Valley (*Qian Gu*, SI 2), Great Mound (*Da Ling*, Per 7), Spring at the Bend (*Qu Quan*, Liv 8), (Arm) Three *Li* (*San Li*, LI 10), Sunken Valley (*Xian Gu*, St 43), Blazing Valley (*Ran Gu*, Ki 2), Moving Between (*Xing Jian*, Liv 2), (Foot) Overlooking Tears (*Lin Qi*, GB 41), and Lung *Shu* (*Fei Shu*, Bl 13)

For counterflow coughing with nothing emitted: First choose (Leg) Three *Li* (*San Li*, St 36) and then choose Supreme White (*Tai Bai*, Sp 3), Liver *Shu* (*Gan Shu*, Bl 18), Great Abyss (*Tai Yuan*, Lu 9), Fish Border (*Yu Ji*, Lu 10), Great Ravine (*Tai Xi*, Ki 3), and (Foot) Portal Yin (*Qiao Yin*, GB 44).

---

3   Running piglet is another name for kidney *ji* or renal accumulation. It is shaped like a piglet lying in the lower abdomen and often sending qi towards the heart or even higher to the throat.

For counterflow coughing and shivering with cold: Lesser Shang (*Shao Shang*, Lu 11) and Celestial Chimney (*Tian Tu*, CV 22) [moxa with 3 cones]

For enduring disease of coughing: Lesser Shang (*Shao Shang*, Lu 11) and Celestial Pillar (*Tian Zhu*, Bl 10) [moxa with 3 cones]

For inverted qi surging into the abdomen[4]: Ravine Divide (*Jie Xi*, St 41) and Celestial Chimney (*Tian Tu*, CV 22)

For shortness of breath: Great Mound (*Da Ling*, Per 7) and Cubit Marsh (*Chi Ze*, Lu 5)

For diminished qi: Intermediary Courier (*Jian Shi*, Per 5), Spirit Gate (*Shen Men*, Ht 7), Great Mound (*Da Ling*, Per 7), Lesser Surge (*Shao Chong*, Ht 9), (Leg) Three *Li* (*San Li*, St 36), Lower Ridge (*Xia Lian*, St 39), Moving Between (*Xing Jian*, Liv 2), Blazing Valley (*Ran Gu*, Ki 2), Reaching Yin (*Zhi Yin*, Bl 67), Lung *Shu* (*Fei Shu*, Bl 13), and Sea of Qi (*Qi Hai*, CV 6)

For yawning qi: Connecting the Interior (*Tong Li*, Ht 5) and Inner Court (*Nei Ting*, St 44)

For various kinds of accumulation: (Leg) Three *Li* (*San Li*, St 36), Yin Valley (*Yin Gu*, Ki 10), Ravine Divide (*Jie Xi*, St 41), Open Valley (*Tong Gu*, Ki 20), Upper Venter (*Shang Wan*, CV 13), Lung *Shu* (*Fei Shu*, Bl 13), Diaphragm *Shu* (*Ge Shu*, Bl 17), Spleen *Shu* (*Pi Shu*, Bl 20), and Triple Heater *Shu* (*San Jiao Shu*, Bl 22)

For qi lumps in the abdomen: One point (should be located) at the head of the lump. Needle this 2.5 *cun* deep (and) moxa it

---

4   Inverted qi is a disorder due to disharmony between yin and yang, chaotic qi and blood, blocking phlegm turbidity, retained food accumulation, or great pain. It may lead to limb frigidity or sudden collapse.

with 2 times 7 cones. One point (should be located) in the center of the lump. Needle (this point) 3 *cun* deep (and) moxa it with 3 times 7 cones. One point (should be located) at the tail of the lump. Needle this 3.5 *cun* deep (and) moxa it with 7 cones.

For chest and abdominal inflating distention and rapid dyspneic breathing: Union Valley (*He Gu*, LI 4), (Arm) Three *Li* (*San Li*, LI 10), Cycle Gate (*Qi Men*, Liv 14), and Breast Root (*Ru Gen*, St 18)

Moxa method for wheezing: Celestial Chimney (*Tian Tu*, CV 22) and the end of the coccyx (*i.e.*, *Chang Qiang*, Long Strong, GV 1). There is also a point on the upper back. The method of locating it (consists of) putting a thread around the neck and hanging it in the front. Cut the thread at the tip of the xiphoid process. Turn the thread around so that its ends are on the spine. The point is at the place where the ends are. Moxa with 7 cones. Its efficacy is untold.

The Category of Abdominal Pain, Distention & Fullness

For abdominal pain: Inner Pass (*Nei Guan*, Per 6), (Leg) Three Li (*San Li*, St 36), Yin Valley (*Yin Gu*, Ki 10), Yin Mound (Spring) (*Yin Ling*, Sp 9), Recover Flow (*Fu Liu*, Ki 7), Great Ravine (*Tai Xi*, Ki 3), Kunlun (Mountain), (*Kun Lun*, Bl 60), Sunken Valley (*Xian Gu*, St 43), Moving Between (*Xing Jian*, Liv 2), Supreme White (*Tai Bai*, Sp 3), Central Venter (*Zhong Wan*, CV 12), Sea of Qi (*Qi Hai*, CV 6), Diaphragm *Shu* (*Ge Shu*, Bl 17), Spleen *Shu* (*Pi Shu*, Bl 20), and Kidney *Shu* (*Shen Shu*, Bl 23)

For inability to ingest: Inner Pass (*Nei Guan*, Per 6), Fish Border (*Yu Ji*, Lu 10), and (Leg) Three Li (*San Li*, St 36)[1]

For unbearable, acute lower abdominal pain, small intestine qi[2], withdrawn external kidneys[3], *shan qi*, and various kinds of qi pain and heart pain: Moxa with 5 cones the midpoint of the crease on the plantar surface of the second phalangeal joint of the toe next to the big one, the left one for males and the right for females. This is miraculous. It is also alright to moxa both feet.

---

[1] Arm Three Li (*Shou San Li*, LI 10) is also effective for digestive disorders and may be implied here.

[2] Small intestine qi is a kind of *shan* characterized by lower abdominal cold pain giving a dragging discomfort to the testicles and lumbus.

[3] In Chinese, the testicles are sometimes known as the external kidneys.

For lower abdominal distending pain: Sea of Qi (*Qi Hai*, CV 6)

For periumbilical pain: Water Divide (*Shui Fen*, CV 9), Spirit Gate (*Shen Que*, CV 8), and Sea of Qi (*Qi Hai*, CV 6)

For lower abdominal pain: Yin Market (*Yin Shi*, St 33), Mountain Support (*Cheng Shan*, Bl 57), Lower Ridge (*Xia Lian*, St 39), Recover Flow (*Fu Liu*, Ki 7), Mound Center (*Zhong Feng*, Liv 4), Great Pile (*Da Dun*, Liv 1), Small Sea (*Xiao Hai*, SI 8), Origin Pass (*Guan Yuan*, CV 4), and Kidney *Shu* (*Shen Shu*, Bl 23) [the same number of cones as years of age]

For pain by the side of the navel: Upper Ridge (*Shang Lian*, St 37)

For umbilical pain: Spring at the Bend (*Qu Quan*, Liv 8), Mound Center (*Zhong Feng*, Liv 4), and Water Divide (*Shui Fen*, CV 9)

For (abdominal pain) resulting in a dragging ache in the lumbus: Supreme Surge (*Tai Chong*, Liv 3) and Supreme White (*Tai Bai*, Sp 3)

For abdominal fullness: Lesser Shang (*Shao Shang*, Lu 11), Yin Market (*Yin Shi*, St 33), (Leg) Three *Li* (*San Li*, St 36), Spring at the Bend (*Qu Quan*, Liv 8), Kunlun (Mountain, *Kun Lun*, Bl 60), Shang Hill (*Shang Qiu*, Sp 5), Valley Passage (*Tong Gu*, Bl 66), Supreme White (*Tai Bai*, Sp 3), Great Metropolis (*Da Du*, Sp 2), Hidden White (*Yin Bai*, Sp 1), Sunken Valley (*Xian Gu*, St 43), and Moving Between (*Xing Jian*, Liv 2)

For abdominal and costal fullness: Yang Mound (Spring) (*Yang Ling*, GB 34), (Leg) Three *Li* (*San Li*, St 36), and Upper Ridge (*Shang Lian*, St 37)

For heart and abdominal distention and fullness: Severed Bone (*Jue Gu*, GB 39) and Inner Court (*Nei Ting*, St 44)

For lower abdominal distention, fullness, and pain: Mound Center (*Zhong Feng*, Liv 4), Blazing Valley (*Ran Gu*, Ki 2), Inner Court (*Nei Ting*, St 44), and Great Pile (*Da Dun*, Liv 1)

For abdominal distention: Cubit Marsh (*Chi Ze*, Lu 5), Yin Market (*Yin Shi*, St 33), (Leg) Three *Li* (*San Li*, St 36), Spring at the Bend (*Qu Quan*, Liv 8), Yin Valley (*Yin Gu*, Ki 10), Yin Mound (Spring) (*Yin Ling*, Sp 9), Shang Hill (*Shang Qiu*, Sp 5), Offspring of the Noble (*Gong Sun*, Sp 4), Inner Court (*Nei Ting*, St 44), Great Ravine (*Tai Xi*, Ki 3), Supreme White (*Tai Bai*, Sp 3), Severe Mouth (*Li Dui*, St 45), Hidden White (*Yin Bai*, Sp 1), Diaphragm *Shu* (*Ge Shu*, Bl 17), Kidney *Shu* (*Shen Shu*, Bl 23), Central Venter (*Zhong Wan*, CV 12), and Large Intestine *Shu* (*Da Chang Shu*, Bl 25)

For stomach distention with ache: Diaphragm *Shu* (*Ge Shu*, Bl 17)

For abdominal hardness and enlargement: (Leg) Three *Li* (*San Li*, St 36), Yin Mound (Spring) (*Yin Ling*, Sp 9), Hill Ruins (*Qiu Xu*, GB 40), Ravine Divide (*Jie Xi*, St 41), Surging Yang (*Chong Yang*, St 42), Cycle Gate (*Qi Men*, Liv 14), Water Divide (*Shui Fen*, CV 9), Spirit Gate (*Shen Que*, CV 8), and Bladder *Shu* (*Pang Guang Shu*, Bl 28)

For (alternating) cold and heat with (abdominal) hardness and enlargement: Surging Yang (*Chong Yang*, St 42)

For drum distention: Recover Flow (*Fu Liu*, Ki 7), Mound Center (*Zhong Feng*, Liv 4), Offspring of the Noble (*Gong Sun*, Sp 4), Supreme White (*Tai Bai*, Sp 3), Water Divide (*Shui Fen*, CV 9), and Three Yin Intersection (*San Yin Jiao*, Sp 6)

For cold abdomen with inability to ingest: Yin Mound Spring (*Yin Ling Quan*, Sp 9) [moxa]

For elusive phlegm[4] abdominal cold: Three Yin Intersection (*San Yin Jiao*, Sp 6)

For rumbling in the abdomen with (alternating) cold and heat: Recover Flow (*Fu Liu*, Ki 7)

For gastric and abdominal inflating distention and qi rumbling: Union Valley (*He Gu*, LI 4), (Leg) Three *Li* (*San Li*, St 36), and Cycle Gate (*Qi Men*, Liv 14)

---

[4] This is phlegm *pi* in Wiseman *et al.*'s terminology. *Pi* means far-removed, distant, obscure, etc. in Chinese. Therefore, elusive phlegm is a recurring mass due to accumulated phlegm.

The Category of Heart, Spleen & Stomach

For heart pain: Marsh at the Bend (*Qu Ze*, Per 3), Intermediary Courier (*Jian Shi*, Per 5), Inner Pass (*Nei Guan*, Per 6), Great Mound (*Da Ling*, Per 7), Spirit Gate (*Shen Men*, Ht 7), Great Abyss (*Tai Yuan*, Lu 9), Great Ravine (*Tai Xi*, Ki 3), Valley Passage (*Tong Gu*, Bl 66), Heart *Shu* (*Xin Shu*, Bl 15) [100 cones], and Great Tower Gate (*Ju Que*, CV 14) [7 cones]

For heart pain with inability to transform food: Central Venter (*Zhong Wan*, CV 12)

For pain in the central venter: Great Abyss (*Tai Yuan*, Lu 9), Fish Border (*Yu Ji*, Lu 10), (Leg) Three *Li* (*San Li*, St 36), the points under the two breasts [1 *cun* below, each 30 cones], Diaphragm *Shu* (*Ge Shu*, Bl 17), Stomach *Shu* (*Wei Shu*, Bl 21), and Kidney *Shu* (*Shen Shu*, Bl 23) [the same number of cones as years of age]

For heart vexation: Spirit Gate (*Shen Men*, Ht 7), Yang Ravine (*Yang Xi*, LI 5), Fish Border (*Yu Ji*, Lu 10), Wrist Bone (*Wan Gu*, SI 4), Lesser Shang (*Shao Shang*, Lu 11), Ravine Divide (*Jie Xi*, St 41), Offspring of the Noble (*Gong Sun*, Sp 4), Supreme White (*Tai Bai*, Sp 3), and Reaching Yin (*Zhi Yin*, Bl 67)

For vexation, thirst, and hot heart: Marsh at the Bend (*Qu Ze*, Per 3)

For vexation and racing of the heart: Fish Border (*Yu Ji*, Lu 10)

For sudden unbearable heart pain and vomiting of cold acid water: Moxa the inner crease of the toe next to the big one, each foot 1 cone the size of a grain of wheat. This gives instantaneous relief.

For excessive thought and worry (resulting in) the heart lacking in strength with forgetfulness: Moxa Hundred Convergences (*Bai Hui*, GV 20).

For heart wind[1]: Heart *Shu* (*Xin Shu*, Bl 15) [moxa] and Central Venter (*Zhong Wan*, CV 12)

For vexation and oppression: Wrist Bone (*Wan Gu*, SI 4)

For vacuity vexation with a dry mouth: Lung *Shu* (*Fei Shu*, Bl 13)

For vexation, oppression, and insomnia: Great Abyss (*Tai Yuan*, Lu 9), Offspring of the Noble (*Gong Sun*, Sp 4), Hidden White (*Yin Bai*, Sp 1), Lung *Shu* (*Fei Shu*, Bl 13), Yin Mound Spring (*Yin Ling Quan*, Sp 9), and Three Yin Intersection (*San Yin Jiao*, Sp 6)

For heart vexation and frequent eructation: Lesser Shang (*Shao Shang*, Lu 11), Great Ravine (*Tai Xi*, Ki 3), and Sunken Valley (*Xian Gu*, St 43)

---

[1] The signs and symptoms of heart wind are spontaneous sweating, aversion to wind, red lips, somnolence, impaired memory, and palpitations. These are due to the intrusion of wind into the heart. There is, however, another kind of heart wind which may also be called internal wind. It is manifested by mental disorders, such as trance, changeable moods, and confused speech.

For heart *bi*[2] with melancholy and apprehension: Spirit Gate (*Shen Men*, Ht 7), Great Mound (*Da Ling*, Per 7), and Fish Border (*Yu Ji*, Lu 10)

For indolence and sluggishness: Shining Sea (*Zhao Hai*, Ki 6)

For the heart fraught with fright and apprehension: Marsh at the Bend (*Qu Ze*, Per 3), Celestial Well (*Tian Jing*, TH 10), Spirit Pathway (*Ling Dao*, Ht 4), Spirit Gate (*Shen Men*, Ht 7), Great Mound (*Da Ling*, Per 7), Fish Border (*Yu Ji*, Lu 10), Second Space (*Er Jian*, LI 2), Humor Gate (*Ye Men*, TH 2), Lesser Surge (*Shao Chong*, Ht 9), Hundred Convergences (*Bai Hui*, GV 20), Severe Mouth (*Li Dui*, St 45), Valley Passage (*Tong Gu*, Bl 66), Great Tower Gate (*Ju Que*, CV 14), and Screen Gate (*Zhang Men*, Liv 13)

For liking to lie down (*i.e.*, lethargy or somnolence): Hundred Convergences (*Bai Hui*, GV 20), Celestial Well (*Tian Jing*, TH 10), Third Space (*San Jian*, LI 3), Second Space (*Er Jian*, LI 2), Great Ravine (*Tai Xi*, Ki 3), Shining Sea (*Zhao Hai*, Ki 6), Severe Mouth (*Li Dui*, St 45), and Liver *Shu* (*Gan Shu*, Bl 18)

For liking to lie down with disinclination to speak: Diaphragm *Shu* (*Ge Shu*, Bl 17)

For insomnia: Great Abyss (*Tai Yuan*, Lu 9), Offspring of the Noble (*Gong Sun*, Sp 4), Hidden White (*Yin Bai*, Sp 1), Lung *Shu* (*Fei Shu*, Bl 13), Yin Mound (Spring) (*Yin Ling*, Sp 9), and Three Yin Intersection (*San Yin Jiao*, Sp 6)

For propping fullness and inability to ingest: Lung *Shu* (*Fei Shu*, Bl 13)

---

[2] Heart *bi*, which is a result of vessel *bi*, manifests mainly with palpitations, chest oppression, vexation and agitation, dyspnea, and heart pain.

For shivering with cold and inability to ingest: Surging Yang (*Chong Yang*, St 42)

For a hot stomach with inability to ingest: Lower Ridge (*Xia Lian*, St 39)

For stomach distention with inability to ingest: Water Divide (*Shui Fen*, CV 9)

For heart trance[3]: Celestial Well (*Tian Jing*, TH 10), Great Tower Gate (*Ju Que*, CV 14), and Heart *Shu* (*Xin Shu*, Bl 15)

For heart laughing (*i.e.*, incessant laughing): Yang Ravine (*Yang Xi*, LI 5), Yang Valley (*Yang Gu*, SI 5), Spirit Gate (*Shen Men*, Ht 7), Great Mound (*Da Ling*, Per 7), Broken Sequence (*Lie Que*, Lu 7), Fish Border (*Yu Ji*, Lu 10), Palace of Toil (*Lao Gong*, Per 8), Recover Flow (*Fu Liu*, Ki 7), and Lung *Shu* (*Fei Shu*, Bl 13)

For stomachache: Great Abyss (*Tai Yuan*, Lu 9), Fish Border (*Yu Ji*, Lu 10), (Leg) Three *Li* (*San Li*, St 36), Kidney *Shu* (*Shen Shu*, Bl 23), Lung *Shu* (*Fei Shu*, Bl 13), Stomach *Shu* (*Wei Shu*, Bl 21), and the points under the two breasts [moxa 1 cun below, each with 21 cones]

For stomach reflux: First choose Lower Venter (*Xia Wan*, CV 10) and then (Leg) Three *Li* (*San Li*, St 36) [drain], Stomach *Shu* (*Wei Shu*, Bl 21), Diaphragm *Shu* (*Ge Shu*, Bl 17) [100 cones], Central Venter (*Zhong Wan*, CV 12), and Spleen *Shu* (*Pi Shu*, Bl 20)

For upper esophageal constriction with food unable to go down: Palace of Toil (*Lao Gong*, Per 8), Lesser Shang (*Shao Shang*, Lu 11), Supreme White (*Tai Bai*, Sp 3), Offspring of the Noble (*Gong*

---

[3] One should note that, in TCM, mental or neurotic disorders are usually ascribed to the heart.

44

Sun, Sp 4), (Leg) Three *Li* (*San Li*, St 36), Central Eminence (*Zhong Kui*, M-UE-16) [at the tip of the second phalangeal joint of the middle finger], Diaphragm *Shu* (*Ge Shu*, Bl 17), Heart *Shu* (*Xin Shu*, Bl 15), Stomach *Shu* (*Wei Shu*, Bl 21), Triple Heater *Shu* (*San Jiao Shu*, Bl 22), Central Venter (*Zhong Wan*, CV 12), and Large Intestine *Shu* (*Da Chang Shu*, Bl 25)

For inability to ingest: Lesser Shang (*Shao Shang*, Lu 11), (Leg) Three *Li* (*San Li*, St 36), Blazing Valley (*Ran Gu*, Ki 2), Diaphragm *Shu* (*Ge Shu*, Bl 17), Stomach *Shu* (*Wei Shu*, Bl 21), and Large Intestine *Shu* (*Da Chang Shu*, Bl 25)

For no desire for food: Mound Center (*Zhong Feng*, Liv 4), Blazing Valley (*Ran Gu*, Ki 2), Inner Court (*Nei Ting*, St 44), Severe Mouth (*Li Dui*, St 45), Hidden White (*Yin Bai*, Sp 1), Yin Mound Spring (*Yin Ling Quan*, Sp 9), Lung *Shu* (*Fei Shu*, Bl 13), Spleen *Shu* (*Pi Shi*, Bl 20), Stomach *Shu* (*Wei Shu*, Bl 21), and Small Intestine *Shu* (*Xiao Chang Shu*, Bl 27)

For (accumulated) food qi with foul smell while eating and drinking: Hundred Convergences (*Bai Hui*, GV 20), Lesser Shang (*Shao Shang*, Lu 11), and (Leg) Three *Li* (*San Li*, St 36). Moxa Chest Center (*Dan Zhong*, CV 17).

For emaciated body in spite of large food intake: Spleen *Shu* (*Pi Shu*, Bl 20) and Stomach *Shu* (*Wei Shu*, Bl 21)

For cold spleen[4]: Third Space (*San Jian*, LI 3), Central Islet (*Zhong Zhu*, TH 3), Humor Gate (*Ye Men*, TH 2), Union Valley (*He Gu*, LI 4), Shang Hill (*Shang Qiu*, Sp 5), Three Yin Intersection (*San Yin Jiao*, Sp 6), Mound Center (*Zhong Feng*, Liv 4), Shining Sea (*Zhao Hai*, Ki 6), Sunken Valley (*Xian Gu*, St 43), Great Ravine

---

[4] Cold spleen is also known as spleen yang vacuity. Its signs and symptoms include abdominal pain, retching and vomiting, diarrhea, and cold limbs.

(*Tai Xi*, Ki 3), Reaching Yin (*Zhi Yin*, Bl 67), and Lumbar *Shu* (*Yao Shu*, GV 2).

For hot stomach[5]: Suspended Bell (*Xuan Zhong*, GB 39)

For cold stomach with existence of phlegm: Diaphragm *Shu* (*Ge Shu*, Bl 17)

For spleen vacuity with abdominal distention and untransformed grains in stools: (Leg) Three *Li* (*San Li*, St 36)

For spleen disease of duck-stool diarrhea: Three Yin Intersection (*San Yin Jiao*, Sp 6)

For spleen vacuity constipation: Shang Hill (*Shang Qiu*, Sp 5) and Three Yin Intersection (*San Yin Jiao*, Sp 6) [30 cones]

For gallbladder vacuity with counterflow retching, (gallbladder) heat, and qi ascension[6]: Sea of Qi (*Qi Hai*, CV 6)

---

[5] The signs and symptoms of hot stomach are a liking for cold drink, halitosis, mouth sores, red gums with liability to bleed, constant hunger, short voiding of scant urine, and dry, bound stools.

[6] Gallbladder vacuity's main manifestations include vacuity vexation and insomnia, palpitations, susceptibility to fright, timidity, and frequent sighing. Often complicated by spleen heat, the signs and symptoms of gallbladder heat are chest oppression, vexation, a bitter taste in the mouth, dry throat, retching of yellow water, dizziness, flowery vision, deafness, ringing in the ears, alternating cold and heat, and, in the extreme, jaundice.

The Category of Heart Evils, Mania & Withdrawal

For heart evil[1] with mania and withdrawal: Bamboo Gathering (*Zan Zhu*, Bl 2), Cubit Marsh (*Chi Ze*, Lu 5), Intermediary Courier (*Jian Shi*, Per 5), and Yang Ravine (*Yang Xi*, LI 5)

For mania and withdrawal: Pool at the Bend (*Qu Chi*, LI 11) [7 cones], Small Sea (*Xiao Hai*, SI 8), Lesser Sea (*Shao Hai*, Ht 3), Intermediary Courier (*Jian Shi*, Per 5), Yang Ravine (*Yang Xi*, LI 5), Yang Valley (*Yang Gu*, SI 5), Great Mound (*Da Ling*, Per 7), Union Valley (*He Gu*, LI 4), Fish Border (*Yu Ji*, Lu 10), Wrist Bone (*Wan Gu*, SI 4), Spirit Gate (*Shen Men*, Ht 7), Humor Gate (*Ye Men*, TH 2), Surging Yang (*Chong Yang*, St 42), Moving Between (*Xing Jian*, Liv 2), and Capital Bone (*Jing Gu*, Bl 64) [moxa all the above], and Lung *Shu* (*Fei Shu*, Bl 13) [100 cones]

For epilepsy: Bamboo Gathering (*Zan Zhu*, Bl 2), Celestial Well (*Tian Jing*, TH 10), Small Sea (*Xiao Hai*, SI 8), Spirit Gate (*Shen Men*, Ht 7), Metal Gate (*Jin Men*, Bl 63), Shang Hill (*Shang Qiu*, Sp 5), Moving Between (*Xing Jian*, Liv 2), Valley Passage (*Tong Gu*, Bl 66), Heart *Shu* (*Xin Shu*, Bl 15) [100 cones], Back Ravine (*Hou Xi*, SI 3), and Ghost Eye (*Gui Yan*) [{*i.e.,*} four points at the inner corners of the nails of the thumbs and big toes. The cones should be set at the juncture between the nail and the flesh. Three cones work wonders.]

---

[1] Heart evil is also known as strike of the heart by ghost evil. This is a mental disorder typically stemming from unidentified causes. It is characterized by sudden onset, confused speech, and confused vision.

For ghost hitting[2]: Intermediary Courier (*Jian Shi*, Per 5) and Branch Ditch (*Zhi Gou*, TH 6)

For madness: Upper Star (*Shang Xing*, GV 23), Hundred Convergences (*Bai Hui*, GV 20), Wind Pool (*Feng Chi*, GB 20), Pool at the Bend (*Qu Chi*, LI 11), Cubit Marsh (*Chi Ze*, Lu 5), Yang Ravine (*Yang Xi*, LI 5), Wrist Bone (*Wan Gu*, SI 4), Ravine Divide (*Jie Xi*, St 41), Back Ravine (*Hou Xi*, SI 3), Extending Vessel (*Shen Mai*, Bl 62), Kunlun (Mountain, *Kun Lun*, Bl 60), Shang Hill (*Shang Qiu*, Sp 5), Blazing Valley (*Ran Gu*, Ki 2), Valley Passage (*Tong Gu*, Bl 66), and Mountain Support (*Cheng Shan*, Bl 57) [needle 3 *fen* deep with quick extraction; moxa with 100 cones]

For maniac speech: Great Abyss (*Tai Yuan*, Lu 9), Yang Ravine (*Yang Xi*, LI 5), Lower Ridge (*Xia Lian*, St 39), and Kunlun (Mountain, *Kun Lun*, Bl 60)

For maniac speech with melancholy: Great Mound (*Da Ling*, Per 7)

For talkativeness: Hundred Convergences (*Bai Hui*, GV 20)

For mania and withdrawal with nonsensical speech whether to superiors or inferiors: Moxa the middle flesh seam inside the lip (*i.e.*, *Yin Jiao*, GV 28) with 1 cone the size of a grain of wheat. It is still better to cut (this seam) with a steel knife.

For maniac speech and frequently looking round: Yang Valley (*Yang Gu*, SI 5) and Humor Gate (*Ye Men*, TH 2)

---

[2] Ghost hitting is similar to heart evil, but it is often ascribed to fright caused by something unexpected. This was believed to be associated with a ghost or devil. In addition, the patient may also complain of seeing or dreaming of ghosts.

For (nervous) laughing: Water Trough (*Shui Gou*, GV 26), Broken Sequence (*Lie Que*, Lu 7), Yang Ravine (*Yang Xi*, LI 5), and Great Mound (*Da Ling*, Per 7)

For laughing and crying (*i.e.*, emotional lability): Hundred Convergences (*Bai Hui*, GV 20) and Water Trough (*Shui Gou*, GV 26)

For maniacally casting one's eyes about: Wind Mansion (*Feng Fu*, GV 16)

For obsession by ghost evils: Intermediary Courier (*Jian Shi*, Per 5). Continue needling with the following 13 points: The first is Ghost Palace (*Gui Gong*, *i.e.*, Human Center, *Ren Zhong*, GV 26). The second is Ghost Sincerity (*Gui Xin*, *i.e.*, Lesser Shang, *Shao Shang*, Lu 11), [near the base of the nail of the thumb; insert {the needle} 3 *fen* deep]. The third is Ghost Pile (*Gui Lei*, *i.e.*, Hidden White, *Yin Bai*, Sp 1), [near the base of the nail of the big toe; insert {the needle} 2 *fen* into the flesh]. The fourth is Ghost Heart (*Gui Xin*, *i.e.*, Great Abyss, *Tai Yuan*, Lu 9). [Insert {the needle} one half *cun* deep. It is unnecessary to needle all these points. No more than 5-6 points will tell. If {the patient's condition} is caused by a supernatural evil spirit, the patient will speak on their own accord the origin {of their condition}. According to past experience, the spirit or sprite may be summoned up instantly, but one need not order them to leave right away. One should begin extracting the needle(s) from the left side in male patients and from the right in female patients. In case a number of points needled should fail to bring effect, needle all (13) points.]

The fifth is Ghost Road (*Gui Lu*, *i.e.*, Extending Vessel, *Shen Mai*, Bl 62); [scour seven times the red-hot needle and use it 2-3 times].[3] The sixth is Ghost Pillow (*Gui Zhen, i.e.,* Wind Mansion, *Feng Fu,* GV 16), [over Great Vertebra {*Da Zhui,* GV 14}, 1 *cun* above the hairline]. The seventh is Ghost Bed (*Gui Chuang, i.e.,* Jawbone, *Jia Che,* St 6), [on the hairline in front of the ears]. The eighth is Ghost Market (*Gui Shi, i.e.,* Sauce Receptacle, *Cheng Jiang,* CV 24]. The ninth is Ghost Palace (*Gui Gong, i.e.,* Palace of Toil, *Lao Gong,* Per 8). The tenth is Ghost Hall (*Gui Tang, i.e.,* Upper Star, *Shang Xing,* GV 23); [scour the red-hot needle seven times]. The eleventh is Ghost Store (*Gui Cang, i.e.,* Meeting of Yin, *Hui Yin,* CV 1), [on the seam of the perineum. Moxa with 3 cones.] The twelfth is Ghost Minister (*Gui Chen, i.e.,* Pool at the Bend, *Qu Chi,* LI 11); [use red-hot needling]. The thirteenth is Ghost Seal (*Gui Feng, i.e.,* Sea Spring, *Hai Quan,* M-HN-37), [on the seam on the undersurface of the tongue 1 *cun* from {its root}]. One should operate at these points in order. The combination of needling and moxaing is the rule.

For seeing ghosts: Yang Ravine (*Yang Xi,* LI 5)

For oppressive ghost dreams: Shang Hill (*Shang Qiu,* Sp 5)

For ghost evil stroke with loss of consciousness: Water Trough (*Shui Gou,* GV 26), Central Venter (*Zhong Wan,* CV 12), and Sea of Qi (*Qi Hai,* CV 6)

For unconsciousness of human affairs: (Leg) Three *Li* (*San Li,* St 36) and Great Pile (*Da Dun,* Liv 1)

For mania: Lesser Sea (*Shao Hai,* Ht 3), Intermediary Courier (*Jian Shi,* Per 5), Spirit Gate (*Shen Men,* Ht 7), Union Valley (*He*

---

[3]   In ancient times, red-hot needling required that the needle be oiled and burnt before use and cleaned after use. Therefore, scouring one time means performing red-hot needling one time. Each needle in each such performance could be used for three points.

Gu, LI 4), Back Ravine (*Hou Xi*, SI 3), Recover Flow (*Fu Liu*, Ki 7), and Silk Bamboo Hole (*Si Zhu Kong*, TH 23)

For mania and withdrawal caused by fascination and obsession with the fox demon[4] and evil god: Tie with a rope the (patient's) big toes and thumbs, moxaing all four places. If any one place is (left) unmoxaed, the illness will never be overcome. Moxa with 3 cones [these are the so-called Ghost Eye {*Gui Yan*} points].

For fetal epilepsy, suckling epilepsy, and fright epilepsy in infants, moxa in the same way with 1 cone the size of a grain of wheat.

For sudden mania: Intermediary Courier (*Jian Shi*, Per 5), Back Ravine (*Hou Xi*, SI 3), and Union Valley (*He Gu*, LI 4)

For maniacal walking: Wind Mansion (*Feng Fu*, GV 16) and Yang Valley (*Yang Gu*, SI 5)

For tugging and slackening and finger contracture: Mute's Gate (*Ya Men*, GV 15), Yang Valley (*Yang Gu*, SI 5), Wrist Bone (*Wan Gu*, SI 4), and Girdling Vessel (*Dai Mai*, GB 26)

For feeble-mindedness: Spirit Gate (*Shen Men*, Ht 7), Lesser Shang (*Shao Shang*, Lu 11), Gushing Spring (*Yong Quan*, Ki 1), and Heart *Shu* (*Xin Shu*, Bl 15)

For enduring mania with climbing heights to sing and running about naked: Spirit Gate (*Shen Men*, Ht 7), Back Ravine (*Hou Xi*, SI 3), and Surging Yang (*Chong Yang*, St 42)

---

4   Fox demons, similar to fox fairies in the English language literature, are types of spirits who enter the soul of a person and strike without notice.

For tugging with fright: Hundred Convergences (*Bai Hui*, GV 20) and Ravine Divide (*Jie Xi*, St 41)

For violent fright: Lower Ridge (*Xia Lian*, St 39)

For madness: Front Valley (*Qian Gu*, SI 2), Back Ravine (*Hou Xi*, SI 3), Water Trough (*Shui Gou*, GV 26), Ravine Divide (*Jie Xi*, St 41), Metal Gate (*Jin Men*, Bl 63), and Extending Vessel (*Shen Mai*, Bl 62)

The Category of Sudden Turmoil
(*i.e.*, Cholera-like Diseases)

F or sudden turmoil: Yin Mound (Spring) (*Yin Ling*, Sp 9), Mountain Support (*Cheng Shan*, Bl 57), Ravine Divide (*Jie Xi*, St 41), and Supreme White (*Tai Bai*, Sp 3)

For sudden turmoil with retching and vomiting: Branch Ditch (*Zhi Gou*, TH 6)

For sudden turmoil with vomiting and diarrhea: Passage Hub (*Guan Chong*, TH 1), Branch Ditch (*Zhi Gou*, TH 6), Cubit Marsh (*Chi Ze*, Lu 5), (Leg) Three *Li* (*San Li*, St 36), and Supreme White (*Tai Bai*, Sp 3). First choose Great Ravine (*Tai Xi*, Ki 3) and then Supreme Granary (*Tai Cang*, *i.e.*, *Zhong Wan*, CV 12).

For sudden turmoil with cramps: Branch Ditch (*Zhi Gou*, TH 6), Passage Hub (*Guan Chong*, TH 1), Yin Mound (Spring) (*Yin Ling*, Sp 9), Mountain Support (*Cheng Shan*, Bl 57), Yang Assistance (*Yang Fu*, GB 38), Mound Center (*Zhong Feng*, Liv 4), Ravine Divide (*Jie Xi*, St 41), Hill Ruins (*Qiu Xu*, GB 40), Offspring of the Noble (*Gong Sun*, Sp 4), Supreme White (*Tai Bai*, Sp 3), and Great Metropolis (*Da Du*, Sp 2)

The Category of Malarial Disease[1]

For malaria: Hundred Convergences (*Bai Hui*, GV 20), Channel Ditch (*Jing Qu*, Lu 8), and Front Valley (*Qian Gu*, SI 2)

For warm malaria[2]: Central Venter (*Zhong Wan*, CV 12) and Great Vertebra (*Da Zhui*, GV 14)

For quartan malaria: Lumbar *Shu* (*Yao Shu*, GV 2)

For malaria with cold and heat: Union Valley (*He Gu*, LI 4), Humor Gate (*Ye Men*, TH 2), and Shang Yang (*Shang Yang*, LI 1)

For phlegm malaria[3] with cold and heat: Back Ravine (*Hou Xi*, SI 3) and Union Valley (*He Gu*, LI 4)

For malaria with quivering with cold: Upper Star (*Shang Xing*,

---

[1] In TCM, malaria may mean the Western medical disease called malaria or may simply refer to diseases characterized by bouts of alternating hot and cold or recurrent fever and chills.

[2] Warm malaria is a disease of exuberant heat due to hidden evils internally and later contraction of summerheat. Its clinical manifestations include heat preceding cold or solely heat without cold following, thirst, liking for cold drink, vexatious aching of the joints of the bones, vomiting in the case of the stomach injured by heat, fatigue, weakness, a red tongue, and a floating, rapid pulse.

[3] Phlegm malaria is a type of malaria complicated by depressive phlegm. Its manifestations, among others, are dizziness, abundant phlegm, counter-flow vomiting, and, in extreme cases, coma.

GV 23), Hill Ruins (*Qiu Xu*, GB 40), and Sunken Valley (*Xian Gu*, St 43)

For headache: Wrist Bone (*Wan Gu*, SI 4)

For cold malaria: Third Space (*San Jian*, LI 3)

For heart vexation: Spirit Gate (*Shen Men*, Ht 7)

For cold malaria with inability to ingest (*i.e.*, lack of appetite): Offspring of the Noble (*Gong Sun*, Sp 4), Inner Court (*Nei Ting*, St 44), and Severe Mouth (*Li Dui*, St 45)

For enduring malaria: Central Islet (*Zhong Zhu*, TH 3), Shang Yang (*Shang Yang*, LI 1), and Hill Ruins (*Qiu Xu*, GB 40)

For more heat than cold: Intermediary Courier (*Jian Shi*, Per 5) and (Leg) Three *Li* (*San Li*, St 36)

For malaria initiated by spleen cold: Great Vertebra (*Da Zhui*, GV 14), Intermediary Courier (*Jian Shi*, Per 5), and Breast Root (*Ru Gen*, St 18)

The Category of Swelling & Distention

F or puffy swelling all over the body: Pool at the Bend (*Qu Chi*, LI 11), Union Valley (*He Gu*, LI 4), (Leg) Three *Li* (*San Li*, St 36), Inner Court (*Nei Ting*, St 44), Moving Between (*Xing Jian*, Liv 2), and Three Yin Intersection (*San Yin Jiao*, Sp 6)

For water swelling: Broken Sequence (*Lie Que*, Lu 7), Wrist Bone (*Wan Gu*, SI 4), Union Valley (*He Gu*, LI 4), Intermediary Courier (*Jian Shi*, Per 5), Yang Mound (Spring) (*Yang Ling*, GB 34), Yin Valley (*Yin Gu*, Ki 10), (Leg) Three *Li* (*San Li*, St 36), Spring at the Bend (*Qu Quan*, Liv 8), Ravine Divide (*Jie Xi*, St 41), Sunken Valley (*Xian Gu*, St 43), Recover Flow (*Fu Liu*, Ki 7), Offspring of the Noble (*Gong Sun*, Sp 4), Severe Mouth (*Li Dui*, St 45), Surging Yang (*Chong Yang*, St 42), Yin Mound (Spring) (*Yin Ling*, Sp 9), Stomach *Shu* (*Wei Shu*, Bl 21), Water Divide (*Shui Fen*, CV 9), and Spirit Gate (*Shen Que*, CV 8)

For puffy swelling of the limbs: Pool at the Bend (*Qu Chi*, LI 11), Connecting the Interior (*Tong Li*, Ht 5), Union Valley (*He Gu*, LI 4), Central Islet (*Zhong Zhu*, TH 3), Humor Gate (*Ye Men*, TH 2), (Leg) Three *Li* (*San Li*, St 36), and Three Yin Intersection (*San Yin Jiao*, Sp 6)

For generalized wind puffy swelling: Ravine Divide (*Jie Xi*, St 41)

For swelling, water qi distention, and fullness: Recover Flow (*Fu Liu*, Ki 7) and Spirit Gate (*Shen Que*, CV 8)

For abdominal lateral costal distention and fullness: Yin Mound Spring (*Yin Ling Quan*, Sp 9)

For generalized swelling and fullness with untransformed food in the stools: Kidney *Shu* (*Shen Shu*, Bl 23) [100 cones]

For drum distention: Recover Flow (*Fu Liu*, Ki 7), Offspring of the Noble (*Gong Sun*, Sp 4), Mound Center (*Zhong Feng*, Liv 4), Supreme White (*Tai Bai*, Sp 3), and Water Divide (*Shui Fen*, CV 9)

For pure-heat wasting thirst: Great Ravine (*Tai Xi*, Ki 3)

For generalized yellowing due to damage by overeating: Screen Gate (*Zhang Men*, Liv 13)

For red jaundice[1]: Hundred Convergences (*Bai Hui*, GV 20), Pool at the Bend (*Qu Chi*, LI 11), Union Valley (*He Gu*, LI 4), (Leg) Three *Li* (*San Li*, St 36), and Bend Middle (*Wei Zhong*, Bl 40)

For jaundice: Hundred Taxations (*Bai Lao*, GV 14), Wrist Bone (*Wan Gu*, SI 4), (Leg) Three *Li* (*San Li*, St 36), Gushing Spring (*Yong Quan*, Ki 1), Central Venter (*Zhong Wan*, CV 12), *Gao Huang (Shu)* (*Gao Huang*, Bl 43), Great Mound (*Da Ling*, Per 7), Palace of Toil (*Lao Gong*, Per 8), Great Ravine (*Tai Xi*, Ki 3), Mound Center (*Zhong Feng*, Liv 4), Blazing Valley (*Ran Gu*, Ki 2), Supreme Surge (*Tai Chong*, Liv 3), Recover Flow (*Fu Liu*, Ki 7), and Spleen *Shu* (*Pi Shu*, Bl 20)

---

[1]   Red jaundice may refer to jaundice accompanied by erythema of the skin.

The Category of Sweating

For copious sweating: First drain Union Valley (*He Gu*, LI 4) and then supplement Recover Flow (*Fu Liu*, Ki 7).

For scant sweating: First supplement Union Valley (*He Gu*, LI 4) and then drain Recover Flow (*Fu Liu*, Ki 7).

For spontaneous sweating: Pool at the Bend (*Qu Chi*, LI 11), Broken Sequence (*Lie Que*, Lu 7), Lesser Shang (*Shao Shang*, Lu 11), Kunlun (Mountain, *Kun Lun*, Bl 60), Surging Yang (*Chong Yang*, St 42), Blazing Valley (*Ran Gu*, Ki 2), Great Pile (*Da Dun*, Liv 1), and Gushing Spring (*Yong Quan*, Ki 1)

For absence of sweating: Upper Star (*Shang Xing*, GV 23), Mute's Gate (*Ya Men*, GV 15), Wind Mansion (*Feng Fu*, GV 16), Wind Pool (*Feng Chi*, GB 20), Branch Ditch (*Zhi Gou*, TH 6), Channel Ditch (*Jing Qu*, Lu 8), Great Mound (*Da Ling*, Per 7), Yang Valley (*Yang Gu*, SI 5), Wrist Bone (*Wan Gu*, SI 4), Blazing Valley (*Ran Gu*, Ki 2), Central Islet (*Zhong Zhu*, TH 3), Humor Gate (*Ye Men*, TH 2), Fish Border (*Yu Ji*, Lu 10), Union Valley (*He Gu*, LI 4), Central Hub (*Zhong Chong*, Per 9), Lesser Shang (*Shao Shang*, Lu 11), Shang Yang (*Shang Yang*, LI 1), Great Metropolis (*Da Du*, Sp 2), Bend Middle (*Wei Zhong*, Bl 40), Sunken Valley (*Xian Gu*, St 43), Severe Mouth (*Li Dui*, St 45), and Pinched Ravine (*Xia Xi*, GB 43)

For sweat refusing to exude: Marsh at the Bend (*Qu Ze*, Per 3), Fish Border (*Yu Ji*, Lu 10), Lesser Marsh (*Shao Ze*, SI 1), Upper Star (*Shang Xing*, GV 23), Spring at the Bend (*Qu Quan*, Liv 8), Recover Flow (*Fu Liu*, Ki 7), Kunlun (Mountain) (*Kun Lun*, Bl 60),

Pinched Ravine (*Xia Xi*, GB 43), and (Foot) Portal Yin (*Qiao Yin*, GB 44)

The Category of *Bi* & Inversion

For wind *bi*[1]: Cubit Marsh (*Chi Ze*, Lu 5) and Yang Assistance (*Yang Fu*, GB 38)

For accumulation *bi* and phlegm *bi*[2]: Diaphragm *Shu* (*Ge Shu*, Bl 17)

For cold inversion[3]: Great Abyss (*Tai Yuan*, Lu 9) and Humor Gate (*Ye Men*, TH 2)

For atonic inversion[4]: Hill Ruins (*Qiu Xu*, GB 40)

For corpse inversion which looks like death with loss of consciousness of human affairs: Moxa Severe Mouth (*Li Dui*, St 45) [3 cones].

For generalized cold *bi*: Pool at the Bend (*Qu Chi*, LI 11), Broken Sequence (*Lie Que*, Lu 7), Jumping Round (*Huan Tiao*, GB 30),

---

[1]   Wind *bi* is characterized by migratory pain of the joints and muscles.

[2]   This entry should be rendered as phlegm accumulation *bi* to make it more understandable. This refers to *bi* complicated by phlegm.

[3]   Cold inversion is often initiated by fatigue, insomnia, hunger, etc. It is due to yang qi vacuity. Its signs and symptoms are aversion to cold, chest and abdominal discomfort, and untransformed grain in the stools, besides limb frigidity. In extreme cases, there may also be collapse.

[4]   Atonic inversion is a combination of atony and inversion patterns. Its symptoms are weakness *and* frigidity of the limbs.

Wind Market (*Feng Shi*, GB 31), Bend Middle (*Wei Zhong*, Bl 40), Shang Hill (*Shang Qiu*, Sp 5), Mound Center (*Zhong Feng*, Liv 4), and (Foot) Overlooking Tears (*Lin Qi*, GB 41)

For counterflow inversion[5]: Yang Assistance (*Yang Fu*, GB 38), (Foot) Overlooking Tears (*Lin Qi*, GB 41), and Screen Gate (*Zhang Men*, Liv 13). In case of an expired pulse, moxa Intermediary Courier (*Jian Shi*, Per 5) or needle Recover Flow (*Fu Liu*, Ki 7).

For corpse inversion: Broken Sequence (*Lie Que*, Lu 7), Central Hub (*Zhong Chong*, Per 9), Metal Gate (*Jin Men*, Bl 63), Great Metropolis (*Da Du*, Sp 2), Inner Court (*Nei Ting*, St 44), Severe Mouth (*Li Dui*, St 45), Hidden White (*Yin Bai*, Sp 1), and Great Pile (*Da Dun*, Liv 1)

For limb inversion: Cubit Marsh (*Chi Ze*, Lu 5), Small Sea (*Xiao Hai*, SI 8), Branch Ditch (*Zhi Gou*, TH 6), Front Valley (*Qian Gu*, SI 2), (Leg) Three *Li* (*San Li*, St 36), Three Yin Intersection (*San Yin Jiao*, Sp 6), Spring at the Bend (*Qu Quan*, Liv 8), Shining Sea (*Zhao Hai*, Ki 6), Great Ravine (*Tai Xi*, Ki 3), Inner Court (*Nei Ting*, St 44), Moving Between (*Xing Jian*, Liv 2), and Great Metropolis (*Da Du*, Sp 2)

---

[5] There are two types of counterflow inversion. One is frigidity of the limbs. The other is violent pain in the chest and abdomen with sudden cold in the feet and a choppy pulse.

The Category of the Intestines, Hemorrhoids & Feces

For rumbling intestines: (Leg) Three *Li* (*San Li*, St 36), Sunken Valley (*Xian Gu*, St 43), Offspring of the Noble (*Gong Sun*, Sp 4), Supreme White (*Tai Bai*, Sp 3), Screen Gate (*Zhang Men*, Liv 13), Three Yin Intersection (*San Yin Jiao*, Sp 6), Water Divide (*Shui Fen*, CV 9), Spirit Gate (*Shen Que*, CV 8), Stomach *Shu* (*Wei Shu*, Bl 21), and Triple Heater *Shu* (*San Jiao Shu*, Bl 22)

For rumbling intestines with diarrhea: Spirit Gate (*Shen Que*, CV 8), Water Divide (*Shui Fen*, CV 9), and Third Space (*San Jian*, LI 3)

For food diarrhea[1]: Upper Ridge (*Shang Lian*, St 37) and Lower Ridge (*Xia Lian*, St 39)

For fulminating diarrhea: Hidden White (*Yin Bai*, Sp 1)

For throughflux diarrhea: Kidney *Shu* (*Shen Shu*, Bl 23)

For duck-stool diarrhea: Supreme Surge (*Tai Chong*, Liv 3), Spirit Gate (*Shen Que*, CV 8), and Three Yin Intersection (*San Yin Jiao*, Sp 6)

For incessant diarrhea: Spirit Gate (*Shen Que*, CV 8)

---

[1] Food diarrhea is due to food damage and is characterized by acid regurgitation and bowel movements immediately following abdominal pain with relief following the movement.

For diarrhea without notice: Central Venter (*Zhong Wan*, CV 12)

For dysentery: Spring at the Bend (*Qu Quan*, Liv 8), Great Ravine (*Tai Xi*, Ki 3), Supreme Surge (*Tai Chong*, Liv 3), Cinnabar Field (*Dan Tian*, i.e., *Guan Yuan*, Origin Pass, CV 4), Spleen *Shu* (*Pi Shu*, Bl 20), and Small Intestine *Shu* (*Xiao Chang Shu*, Bl 27)

For blood in stools: Mountain Support (*Cheng Shan*, Bl 57), Recover Flow (*Fu Ling*, Ki 7), Supreme Surge (*Tai Chong*, Liv 3), and Supreme White (*Tai Bai*, Sp 3)

For fecal incontinence: Cinnabar Field (*Dan Tian*, i.e., *Guan Yuan*, Origin Pass, CV 4) and Large Intestine *Shu* (*Da Chang Shu*, Bl 25)

For constipation: Mountain Support (*Cheng Shan*, Bl 57), Great Ravine (*Tai Xi*, Ki 3), Shining Sea (*Zhao Hai*, Ki 6), Supreme Surge (*Tai Chong*, Liv 3), Small Intestine *Shu* (*Xiao Chang Shu*, Bl 27), Supreme White (*Tai Bai*, Sp 3), Screen Gate (*Zhang Men*, Liv 13), and Bladder *Shu* (*Pang Guang Shu*, Bl 28)

For rectal pressure: Mountain Support (*Cheng Shan*, Bl 57), Ravine Divide (*Jie Xi*, St 41), Supreme White (*Tai Bai*, Sp 3), and Girdling Vessel (*Dai Mai*, GB 26)

For fecal block: Shining Sea (*Zhao Hai*, Ki 6), Supreme White (*Tai Bai*, Sp 3), and Screen Gate (*Zhang Men*, Liv 13)

For diarrhea and loose bowels: Spring at the Bend (*Qu Quan*, Liv 8), Yin Mound (Spring) (*Yin Ling*, Sp 9), Blazing Valley (*Ran Gu*, Ki 2), Bundle Bone (*Shu Gu*, Bl 65), Hidden White (*Yin Bai*, Sp 1), Triple Heater *Shu* (*San Jiao Shu*, Bl 22), Central Venter (*Zhong Wan*, CV 12), Celestial Pivot (*Tian Shu*, St 25), Spleen *Shu* (*Pi Shu*, Bl 20), Kidney *Shu* (*Shen Shu*, Bl 23), and Large Intestine *Shu* (*Da Chang Shu*, Bl 25)

For the five kinds of hemorrhoids[2]: Bend Middle (*Wei Zhong*, Bl 40), Mountain Support (*Cheng Shan*, Bl 57), Taking Flight (*Fei Yang*, Bl 58), Yang Assistance (*Yang Fu*, GB 38), Recover Flow (*Fu Liu*, Ki 7), Supreme Surge (*Tai Chong*, Liv 3), Pinched Ravine (*Xia Xi*, GB 43), Sea of Qi (*Qi Hai*, CV 6), Meeting of Yin (*Hui Yin*, CV 1), and Long Strong (*Chang Qiang*, GV 1)

For intestinal wind[3]: Moxa the end of the coccyx with 100 cones and there will be an immediate cure.

For urinary and fecal stoppage: Stomach Venter (*Wei Wan*, *i.e.*, *Zhong Wan*, Center Venter, CV 12) [moxa 300 cones]

For intestinal *yong*[4] with pain: Supreme White (*Tai Bai*, Sp 3), Sunken Valley (*Xian Gu*, St 43), and Large Intestine *Shu* (*Da Chang Shu*, Bl 25)

For prolapse of the rectum: Hundred Convergences (*Bai Hui*, GV 20), Tail Bone (*Wei Lu*, *i.e.*, *Chang Jiang*, Long Strong, GV 1) [7

---

2   *I.e.*, masculine piles, feminine piles, intestinal piles, vessel(-like) piles, and bloody piles. Masculine piles refer to the growth of fistulas around the anus that often issue forth bloody pus. Feminine piles refer to swelling around the anus. Intestinal piles are a painful swelling with a hard core around the anus which issues forth blood. They are accompanied by cold and heat. Vessel(-like) piles refer to anal fissures. And bloody piles refer to piles with copious bleeding.

3   If wind and heat or dampness and heat are in conflict in the intestines, the connecting vessels there may be damaged. In that case, there will be copious blood in the stools. This is so-called intestinal wind.

4   The signs and symptoms of intestinal *yong* include acute lower abdominal pain which is exacerbated by pressure, a liking for lying down in a curled, recumbent position, cold and heat, and nausea and diarrhea or constipation.

cones] and Navel Center (*Qi Zhong, i.e., Shen Que,* Spirit Gate, CV 8) [the same number of cones as years of age]

For bloody pile diarrhea[5] with abdominal pain: Mountain Support (*Cheng Shan,* Bl 57) and Recover Flow (*Fu Liu,* Ki 7)

For hemorrhoids and bone *ju* erosion[6]: Mountain Support (*Cheng Shan,* Bl 57) and Shang Hill (*Shang Qiu,* Sp 5)

For enduring piles: Two Whites (*Er Bai,* M-UE-29) [4 *cun* proximal to the palm], Mountain Support (*Cheng Shan,* Bl 57), and Long Strong (*Chang Qiang,* GV 1)

---

[5]   Bloody pile diarrhea refers to diarrhea accompanying piles and is characterized by rectal pressure and bleeding.

[6]   Lesions deep enough to affect the bone are called bone *ju* erosion.

The Category of the Genitals, *Shan* & Urination

For cold *shan* abdominal pain[1]: Yin Market (*Yin Shi*, St 33), Great Ravine (*Tai Xi*, Ki 3), and Liver *Shu* (*Gan Shu*, Bl 18)

For *shan* conglomeration[2]: Yin Motility (*Yin Qiao*, Ki 6). [These two points are located in the depressions under the inner malleoli. They are the ruling points for sudden *shan* with lower abdominal pain. Choose the right point for conditions on the left side and choose the left point for conditions on the right side. Moxa with 3 cones. For menstrual irregularities in women, also moxa these.]

For sudden *shan*: Hill Ruins (*Qiu Xu*, GB 40), Great Pile (*Da Dun*, Liv 1), Yin Market (*Yin Shi*, St 33), and Shining Sea (*Zhao Hai*, Ki 6)

For *tui shan*[3]: Spring at the Bend (*Qu Quan*, Liv 8), Mound Center (*Zhong Feng*, Liv 4), Supreme Surge (*Tai Chong*, Liv 3), and Shang Hill (*Shang Qiu*, Sp 5)

---

[1] Cold *shan* abdominal pain is caused by retention of cold in the abdomen. It is a type of periumbilical pain accompanied by retching and vomiting, massive sweating, and frigidity of the extremities.

[2] *Shan* conglomeration is a kind of *shan* characterized by hot pain in the lower abdomen and whitish, turbid urine.

[3] *Tui shan* refers to a swollen scrotum and enlarged testicles with distention and a sensation of heaviness. It may or may not cause pain or itching.

For bowstring and elusive masses [pain in the lowermost abdomen]: Great Ravine (*Tai Xi*, Ki 3), (Leg) Three *Li* (*San Li*, St 36), Yin Mound (Spring) (*Yin Ling*, Sp 9), Spring at the Bend (*Qu Quan*, Liv 8), Spleen *Shu* (*Pi Shu*, Bl 20), and Three Yin Intersection (*San Yin Jiao*, Sp 6)

For *shan* conglomeration: Yin Mound (Spring) (*Yin Ling*, Sp 9), Great Ravine (*Tai Xi*, Ki 3), Hill Ruins (*Qiu Xu*, GB 40), and Shining Sea (*Zhao Hai*, Ki 6)

For intestinal *pi*, *kui shan*[4], and pain of the small intestine: Open Valley (*Tong Gu*, Ki 20) [moxa 100 cones], Bundle Bone (*Shu Gu*, Bl 65), and Large Intestine *Shu* (*Da Chang Shu*, Bl 25)

For unilateral sagging wooden kidney[5]: Return (*Gui Lai*, St 29), Great Pile (*Da Dun*, Liv 1), and Three Yin Intersection (*San Yin Jiao*, Sp 6)

For yin *shan*[6]: Supreme Surge (*Tai Chong*, Liv 3) and Great Pile (*Da Dun*, Liv 1)

For bowstring and elusive masses in the bladder and small intestine: Perform red-hot needling at Fifth Pivot (*Wu Shu*, GB 27), Sea of Qi (*Qi Hai*, CV 6), (Leg) Three *Li* (*San Li*, St 36), Three

---

4   Intestinal *pi* refers to massive hemafecia. *Kui shan* may mean *tui shan*, but sometimes it refers to a swollen scrotum with ulceration or prolapse of the uterus in women.

5   Wooden kidney refers to insensitive testicles, and sagging refers to a sensation of heaviness.

6   *Yin shan* may be a recurrent lower abdominal pain radiating to the genitals as a result of cold attacking or it may refer to a pain in the testicles radiating to the lower abdomen.

Yin Intersection (*San Yin Jiao*, Sp 6), and Qi Door (*Qi Men*, M-CA-15) [100 cones].

For (one) large and (one) small external kidney with frequent evacuation of stools and frequent voiding of urine, or the testicles withdrawn into the abdomen: Great Pile (*Da Dun*, Liv 1)

For swollen genitals: Spring at the Bend (*Qu Quan*, Liv 8), Great Ravine (*Tai Xi*, Ki 3), Great Pile (*Da Dun*, Liv 1), Kidney *Shu* (*Shen Shu*, Bl 23), and Three Yin Intersection (*San Yin Jiao*, Sp 6)

For pain of the penis: Yin Mound (Spring) (*Yin Ling*, Sp 9), Spring at the Bend (*Qu Quan*, Liv 8), Moving Between (*Xing Jian*, Liv 2), Supreme Surge (*Tai Chong*, Liv 3), Yin Valley (*Yin Gu*, Ki 10), Three Yin Intersection (*San Yin Jiao*, Sp 6), Great Pile (*Da Dun*, Liv 1), Great Ravine (*Tai Xi*, Ki 3), Kidney *Shu* (*Shen Shu*, Bl 23), and Central Pole (*Zhong Ji*, CV 3)

For pain in the penis and wet genitals with sweating: Great Ravine (*Tai Xi*, Ki 3), Fish Border (*Yu Ji*, Lu 10), Central Pole (*Zhong Ji*, CV 3), and Three Yin Intersection (*San Yin Jiao*, Sp 6)

For fetus pressing on the bladder with inability to void urine and dribbling urinary block: Origin Pass (*Guan Yuan*, CV 4)

For kidney viscus vacuity cold, increasing emaciation, taxation damage, terrific pain in the genitals, diminished qi, and seminal emission: Kidney *Shu* (*Shen Shu*, Bl 23)

For seminal emission and white turbidity: Kidney *Shu* (*Shen Shu*, Bl 23), Origin Pass (*Guan Yuan*, CV 4), and Three Yin Intersection (*San Yin Jiao*, Sp 6)

For dream emission and loss of essence: Spring at the Bend (*Qu Quan*, Liv 8) [100 cones], Mound Center (*Zhong Feng*, Liv 4),

Supreme Surge (*Tai Chong*, Liv 3), Reaching Yin (*Zhi Yin*, Bl 67), Diaphragm *Shu* (*Ge Shu*, Bl 17), Spleen *Shu* (*Pi Shu*, Bl 20), Three Yin Intersection (*San Yin Jiao*, Sp 6), Kidney *Shu* (*Shen Shu*, Bl 23), Origin Pass (*Guan Yuan*, CV 4), and Triple Heater *Shu* (*San Jiao Shu*, Bl 22)

For qi dribbling urinary block with cold and heat: Yin Mound Spring (*Yin Ling Quan*, Sp 9)

For dribbling urinary block: Spring at the Bend (*Qu Quan*, Liv 8), Blazing Valley (*Ran Gu*, Ki 2), Yin Mound (Spring) (*Yin Ling*, Sp 9), Moving Between (*Xing Jian*, Liv 2), Great Pile (*Da Dun*, Liv 1), Small Intestine *Shu* (*Xiao Chang Shu*, Bl 27), Gushing Spring (*Yong Quan*, Ki 1), and Qi Door (*Qi Men*, M-CA-15) [100 cones]

For yellow or red (*i.e.*, dark-colored) urine: Yin Valley (*Yin Gu*, Ki 10), Great Ravine (*Tai Xi*, Ki 3), Kidney *Shu* (*Shen Shu*, Bl 23), Sea of Qi (*Qi Hai*, CV 6), Bladder *Shu* (*Pang Guang Shu*, Bl 28), and Origin Pass (*Guan Yuan*, CV 4)

For urine of five colors: Bend Middle (*Wei Zhong*, Bl 40) and Front Valley (*Qian Gu*, SI 2)

For urinary incontinence: Sauce Receptacle (*Cheng Jiang*, CV 24), Yin Mound (Spring) (*Yin Ling*, Sp 9), Bend Middle (*Wei Zhong*, Bl 40), Supreme Surge (*Tai Chong*, Liv 3), Bladder *Shu* (*Pang Guang Shu*, Bl 28), and Great Pile (*Da Dun*, Liv 1)

For urine red like blood: Great Mound (*Da Ling*, Per 7) and Origin Pass (*Guan Yuan*, CV 4)

For fetus pressing on the bladder with inhibited voiding of urine in women: Moxa Origin Pass (*Guan Yuan*, CV 4) [2 times 7 cones].

For enuresis: Spirit Gate (*Shen Men*, Ht 7), Fish Border (*Yu Ji*, Lu 10), Supreme Surge (*Tai Chong*, Liv 3), Great Pile (*Da Dun*, Liv 1), and Origin Pass (*Guan Yuan*, CV 4)

For impotence with testicles withdrawn: Yin Valley (*Yin Gu*, Ki 10), Yin Intersection (*Yin Jiao*, CV 7), Blazing Valley (*Ran Gu*, Ki 2), Mound Center (*Zhong Feng*, Liv 4), and Supreme Surge (*Tai Chong*, Liv 3)

For vaginal protrusion: Supreme Surge (*Tai Chong*, Liv 3), Lesser Mansion (*Shao Fu*, Ht 8), Shining Sea (*Zhao Hai*, Ki 6), and Spring at the Bend (*Qu Quan*, Liv 8)

For unilateral sagging (of the scrotum) in *shan qi*: Use a short thread to measure the distance between the two corners of the patient's mouth. Make the thread of this length into a triangle. With one angle set at the center of the navel, place the other two lateral and inferior to the navel. Two points are thus obtained at these two angles. Moxa the right for disease of the left, and moxa the left for disease of the right. Two times 7 cones offers an instant cure. It is also alright to moxa both points.

For bladder qi attacking the lateral costal and infraumbilical regions with the external kidneys withdrawn into the abdomen: Moxa the points 6 *cun* below and 1 *cun* lateral to the navel, the cones being the size of grains of wheat. Moxa the right for disease of the left, and moxa the left for disease of the right.

The Category of Head & Face

For headache: Hundred Convergences (*Bai Hui*, GV 20), Upper Star (*Shang Xing*, GV 23), Wind Mansion (*Feng Fu*, GV 16), Wind Pool (*Feng Chi*, GB 20), Bamboo Gathering (*Zan Zhu*, Bl 2), Silk Bamboo Hole (*Si Zhu Kong*, TH 23), Small Sea (*Xiao Hai*, SI 8), Yang Ravine (*Yang Xi*, LI 5), Great Mound (*Da Ling*, Per 7), Back Ravine (*Hou Xi*, SI 3), Union Valley (*He Gu*, LI 4), Wrist Bone (*Wan Gu*, SI 4), Central Hub (*Zhong Chong*, Per 9), Central Islet (*Zhong Zhu*, TH 3), Kunlun (Mountain, *Kun Lun*, Bl 60), and Yang Mound (Spring) (*Yang Ling*, GB 34)

For rigidity and ache of the head: Jawbone (*Jia Che*, St 6), Wind Pool (*Feng Chi*, GB 20), Shoulder Well (*Jian Jing*, GB 21), Lesser Sea (*Shao Hai*, Ht 3), Back Ravine (*Hou Xi*, SI 3), and Front Valley (*Qian Gu*, SI 2)

For hemilateral headache: Head Corner (*Tou Wei*, St 8)

For brain abscess[1]: Fontanel Meeting (*Xin Hui*, GV 22) and Valley Passage (*Tong Gu*, Bl 66)

For head wind[2]: Upper Star (*Shang Xing*, GV 23), Before the Vertex (*Qian Ding*, GV 21), Hundred Convergences (*Bai Hui*, GV 20), Yang Valley (*Yang Gu*, SI 5), Union Valley (*He Gu*, LI 4),

---

[1] Brain abscess is translated as nasal sink or deep-source nasal congestion by Wiseman, *et al*.

[2] Head wind is a severe continual headache. It may be either one-sided or both-sided. It usually starts suddenly and, when extreme, affects the eyes.

73

Passage Hub (*Guan Chong*, TH 1), Kunlun (Mountain, *Kun Lun*, Bl 60), and Pinched Ravine (*Xia Xi*, GB 43)

For pain in the brain: Upper Star (*Shang Xing*, GV 23), Wind Pool (*Feng Chi*, GB 20), Brain Hollow (*Nao Kong*, GB 19), Celestial Pillar (*Tian Zhu*, Bl 10), and Lesser Sea (*Shao Hai*, Ht 3)

For head wind with red eyes and face: Connecting the Interior (*Tong Li*, Ht 5) and Ravine Divide (*Jie Xi*, St 41)

For head wind sending a pain to the top of the head: Upper Star (*Shang Xing*, GV 23), Hundred Convergences (*Bai Hui*, GV 20), and Union Valley (*He Gu*, LI 4)

For ambilateral and hemilateral head wind: Hundred Convergences (*Bai Hui*, GV 20), Before the Vertex (*Qian Ding*, GV 21), Spirit Court (*Shen Ting*, GV 24), Upper Star (*Shang Xing*, GV 23), Silk Bamboo Hole (*Si Zhu Kong*, TH 23), Wind Pool (*Feng Chi*, GB 20), Union Valley (*He Gu*, LI 4), Bamboo Gathering (*Zan Zhu*, Bl 2), and Head Corner (*Tou Wei*, St 8)

For head wind following intoxication: Hall of Impression (*Yin Tang*, M-HN-3), Bamboo Gathering (*Zan Zhu*, Bl 2), and (Leg) Three *Li* (*San Li*, St 36)

For head wind with dizziness: Union Valley (*He Gu*, LI 4), Bountiful Bulge (*Feng Long*, St 40), Ravine Divide (*Jie Xi*, St 41), and Wind Pool (*Feng Chi*, GB 20). Moxa (the points on the thighs) in the tiger's mouth (*i.e.*, the region between the 1st and 2nd metacarpal bones) with (the patient's) hands hanging at the legs.

For swollen face: Water Trough (*Shui Gou*, GV 26), Upper Star (*Shang Xing*, GV 23), Bamboo Gathering (*Zan Zhu*, Bl 2), Branch Ditch (*Zhi Gou*, TH 6), Intermediary Courier (*Jian Shi*, Per 5), Central Islet (*Zhong Zhu*, TH 3), Humor Gate (*Ye Men*, TH 2),

Ravine Divide (*Jie Xi*, St 41), Moving Between (*Xing Jian*, Liv 2), Severe Mouth (*Li Dui*, St 45), Yi Xi (*Yi Xi*, Bl 45), Celestial Window (*Tian You*, TH 16), and Wind Pool (*Feng Chi*, GB 20)

For itching and swelling of the face: Welcome Fragrance (*Ying Xiang*, LI 20) and Union Valley (*He Gu*, LI 4)

For ache of both the head and the nape of the neck: Hundred Convergences (*Bai Hui*, GV 20), Behind the Vertex (*Hou Ding*, GV 19), and Union Valley (*He Gu*, LI 4)

For head wind with tearing on exposure to cold: Bamboo Gathering (*Zan Zhu*, Bl 2) and Union Valley (*He Gu*, LI 4)

For headache (accompanied by) rigidity and heaviness of the nape of the neck with inability to raise (the head), arch-backed rigidity, and inability to look about: Sauce Receptacle (*Cheng Jiang*, CV 24) [first supplement and then drain] and Wind Mansion (*Feng Fu*, GV 16)

For clouded head and red eyes: Bamboo Gathering (*Zan Zhu*, Bl 2)

For spinning head: Eye Window (*Mu Chuang*, GB 16), Hundred Convergences (*Bai Hui*, GV 20), Extending Vessel (*Shen Mai*, Bl 62), Reaching Yin (*Zhi Yin*, Bl 67), and Declining Connection (*Luo Que*, Bl 8)

For a swollen face with rigidity of the nape of the neck and nasal polyps: Sauce Receptacle (*Cheng Jiang*, CV 24) [3 *fen* deep; insert (the needle) upward, then downward]

For swelling of the head: Upper Star (*Shang Xing*, GV 23), Before the Vertex (*Qian Ding*, GV 21), Great Mound (*Da Ling*, Per 7) [bleed], and Offspring of the Noble (*Gong Sun*, Sp 4)

For swollen cheek: Jawbone (*Jia Che*, St 6)

For swelling in the jowl and submandibular region: Yang Valley (*Yang Gu*, SI 5), Wrist Bone (*Wan Gu*, SI 4), Front Valley (*Qian Gu*, SI 2), Shang Yang (*Shang Yang*, LI 1), Hill Ruins (*Qiu Xu*, GB 40), Pinched Ravine (*Xia Xi*, GB 43), and Arm Three Li (*Shou San Li*, LI 10)

For wind moving giving a wriggling sensation (in the flesh): Welcome Fragrance (*Ying Xiang*, LI 20)

For hypertonicity of the neck: Wind Mansion (*Feng Fu*, GV 16)

For puffy swelling of the head and eyes: Eye Window (*Mu Chuang*, GB 16) and Sunken Valley (*Xian Gu*, St 43)

For twitching of the eyelids: Head Corner (*Tou Wei*, St 8) and Bamboo Gathering (*Zan Zhu*, Bl 2)

For brain wind[3] with pain: Lesser Sea (*Shao Hai*, Ht 3)

For heavy-headedness and body heat (*i.e.*, generalized fever): Kidney *Shu* (*Shen Shu*, Bl 23)

For supraorbital bone pain: Liver *Shu* (*Gan Shu*, Bl 18)

For brittle and falling hair: Lower Ridge (*Xia Lian*, LI 8)

For floating swelling (*i.e.*, a puffy, swollen face): Severe Mouth (*Li Dui*, St 45)

For swollen face: Moxa Water Divide (*Shui Fen*, CV 9).

---

[3]   Brain wind is a kind of head wind with aversion of the nape and the upper back to cold, and severe cold and ache in the head.

For head and visual spinning with pain and swelling of the skin growing white scales: Moxa Fontanel Meeting (*Xin Hui*, GV 22).

The Category of the Pharynx & Larynx

For throat *bi*[1]: Jawbone (*Jia Che*, St 6), Union Valley (*He Gu*, LI 4), Lesser Shang (*Shao Shang*, Lu 11), Cubit Marsh (*Chi Ze*, Lu 5), Channel Ditch (*Jing Qu*, Lu 8), Yang Ravine (*Yang Xi*, LI 5), Great Mound (*Da Ling*, Per 7), Second Space (*Er Jian*, LI 2), and Front Valley (*Qian Gu*, SI 2)

For chattering of the jaws: Lesser Shang (*Shao Shang*, Lu 11)

For a sensation of something stuck in the throat: Intermediary Courier (*Jian Shi*, Per 5) and Third Space (*San Jian*, LI 3)

For swelling in the throat: Central Islet (*Zhong Zhu*, TH 3) and Great Ravine (*Tai Xi*, Ki 3)

For swelling outside the throat: Humor Gate (*Ye Men*, TH 2)

For inability to swallow down food: Moxa Chest Center (*Dan Zhong*, CV 17).

For throat blockage: Pool at the Bend (*Qu Chi*, LI 11) and Union Valley (*He Gu*, LI 4)

For throat swelling, pain, and blockage allowing no water or grain to come down: Union Valley (*He Gu*, LI 4) and Lesser

---

[1] Throat *bi* refers to a moderate pattern of sore throat with slight swelling and difficulty in swallowing. In most cases, it is chronic, advancing slowly and in an unthreatening manner.

Shang (*Shao Shang*, Lu 11). Simultaneously, prick with a three-edged needle three points in a line on the dorsal aspect of the thumb, at the nail root distal to its first phalangeal joint.

For double moth[2]: Jade Humor (*Yu Ye*, M-HN-20a), Gold Liquid (*Jin Jing*, M-HN-20b), and Lesser Shang (*Shao Shang*, Lu 11)

For single moth: Lesser Shang (*Shao Shang*, Lu 11), Union Valley (*He Gu*, LI 4), and Ridge Spring (*Lian Quan*, CV 23)

For severe throat swelling and blockage: Hide a thin three-edged needle in the tip of a writing brush. While casually pretending to dab Myrrha (*Mo Yao*) with the brush, prick the swollen, blocked place. The patient may otherwise be terrified and cannot be cured.

For sore throat: Wind Mansion (*Feng Fu*, GV 16)

---

[2] Moth, also known as baby moth, refers to a moth-shaped swelling on the side of the pharynx. It may be a solitary or double growth. It causes pain and issues forth a whitish yellow pus because of festering. It may possibly be accompanied by high fever, headache, aversion to cold, etc. This traditional Chinese disease category corresponds to acute tonsillitis in modern Western medicine.

The Category of the Ears & Eyes

F or ringing in the ears: Hundred Convergences (*Bai Hui*, GV 20), Auditory Palace (*Ting Gong*, SI 19), Auditory Convergence (*Ting Hui*, GB 2), Ear Gate (*Er Men*, TH 21), Declining Connection (*Luo Que*, Bl 8), Yang Ravine (*Yang Xi*, LI 5), Yang Valley (*Yang Gu*, SI 5), Front Valley (*Qian Gu*, SI 2), Back Ravine (*Hou Xi*, SI 3), Wrist Bone (*Wan Gu*, SI 4), Central Islet (*Zhong Zhu*, TH 3), Humor Gate (*Ye Men*, TH 2), Shang Yang (*Shang Yang*, LI 1), and Kidney *Shu* (*Shen Shu*, Bl 23)

For purulent ear with sores and liquid pus: Ear Gate (*Er Men*, TH 21), Wind Screen (*Yi Feng*, TH 17), and Union Valley (*He Gu*, LI 4)

For hearing impaired to the degree of deafness: Ear Gate (*Er Men*, TH 21), Wind Pool (*Feng Chi*, GB 20), Pinched Ravine (*Xia Xi*, GB 43), Wind Screen (*Yi Feng*, TH 17), Auditory Convergence (*Ting Hui*, GB 2), and Auditory Palace (*Ting Gong*, SI 19)

For red eyes: Eye Window (*Mu Chuang*, GB 16), Great Mound (*Da Ling*, Per 7), Union Valley (*He Gu*, LI 4), Humor Gate (*Ye Men*, TH 2), Upper Star (*Shang Xing*, GV 23), Bamboo Gathering (*Zan Zhu*, Bl 2), and Silk Bamboo Hole (*Si Zhu Kong*, TH 23)

For eye wind[1] with reddening and ulceration (of the eyes): Yang Valley (*Yang Gu*, SI 5)

---

[1] Eye wind refers to wind evils that have invaded the brain to affect the eyes.

For red screen in the eye: Bamboo Gathering (*Zan Zhu*, Bl 2), Back Ravine (*Hou Xi*, SI 3), and Humor Gate (*Ye Men*, TH 2)

For red eyes with screens: Great Abyss (*Tai Yuan*, Lu 9), Pinched Ravine (*Xia Xi*, GB 43), Bamboo Gathering (*Zan Zhu*, Bl 2), and Wind Pool (*Feng Chi*, GB 20)

For thick eye screen: Union Valley (*He Gu*, LI 4), (Head) Overlooking Tears (*Lin Qi*, GB 15), Angle Vertex (*Jiao Sun*, TH 20), Humor Gate (*Ye Men*, TH 2), Back Ravine (*Hou Xi*, SI 3), Central Islet (*Zhong Zhu*, TH 3), and Bright Eyes (*Jing Ming*, Bl 1)

For white eye screen: (Head) Overlooking Tears (*Lin Qi*, GB 15) and Liver *Shu* (*Gan Shu*, Bl 18)

For eyeball pain: Inner Court (*Nei Ting*, St 44) and Upper Star (*Shang Xing*, GV 23)

For cold tearing[2]: Bright Eyes (*Jing Ming*, Bl 1), (Head) Overlooking Tears (*Lin Qi*, GB 15), Wind Pool (*Feng Chi*, GB 20), and Wrist Bone (*Wan Gu*, SI 4)

For tearing on exposure to wind: Head Corner (*Tou Wei*, St 8), Bright Eyes (*Jing Ming*, Bl 1), (Head) Overlooking Tears (*Lin Qi*, GB 15), and Wind Pool (*Feng Chi*, GB 20)

For eye tearing: (Head) Overlooking Tears (*Lin Qi*, GB 15), Hundred Convergences (*Bai Hui*, GV 20), Humor Gate (*Ye Men*, TH 2), Back Ravine (*Hou Xi*, SI 3), Front Valley (*Qian Gu*, SI 2), and Liver *Shu* (*Gan Shu*, Bl 18)

---

[2]   Cold tearing means tearing on exposure to cold which is worse in winter.

For (eye) screen growing because of wind with unbearable pain in the eyes: Bright Eyes (*Jing Ming*, Bl 1). (Also) moxa the prominence at the base joint of the middle finger with 3 cones.

For ingrown eyelash: Silk Bamboo Hole (*Si Zhu Kong*, TH 23)

For clear-eye blindness: Liver *Shu* (*Gan Shu*, Bl 18) and Shang Yang (*Shang Yang*, LI 1) [Choose the right point for the left eye, and choose the left point for the right eye.]

For acute pain of the canthi of the eyes: Third Space (*San Jian*, LI 3)

For clouded eyes: Head Corner (*Tou Wei*, St 8), Bamboo Gathering (*Zan Zhu*, Bl 2), Bright Eyes (*Jing Ming*, Bl 1), Eye Window (*Mu Chuang*, GB 16), Hundred Convergences (*Bai Hui*, GV 20), Wind Mansion (*Feng Fu*, GV 16), Wind Pool (*Feng Chi*, GB 20), Union Valley (*He Gu*, LI 4), Liver *Shu* (*Gan Shu*, Bl 18), Kidney *Shu* (*Shen Shu*, Bl 23), and Silk Bamboo Hole (*Si Zhu Kong*, TH 23)

For visual dizziness: (Head) Overlooking Tears (*Lin Qi*, GB 15), Wind Mansion (*Feng Fu*, GV 16), Wind Pool (*Feng Chi*, GB 20), Yang Valley (*Yang Gu*, SI 5), Central Islet (*Zhong Zhu*, TH 3), Humor Gate (*Ye Men*, TH 2), Fish Border (*Yu Ji*, Lu 10), and Silk Bamboo Hole (*Si Zhu Kong*, TH 23)

For eye pain: Yang Ravine (*Yang Xi*, LI 5), Second Space (*Er Jian*, LI 2), Great Mound (*Da Ling*, Per 7), Third Space (*San Jian*, LI 3), Front Valley (*Qian Gu*, SI 2), and Upper Star (*Shang Xing*, GV 23)

For wind eyelid-rim ulceration and tearing on exposure to wind: Head Corner (*Tou Wei*, St 8) and Cheek Bone-Hole (*Quan Liao*, SI 18)

For itching and pain in the eye: Bright Light (*Guang Ming*, GB 37) [drain] and Fivefold Confluence (*Wu Hui*, *i.e.*, Hundred Convergences, *Bai Hui*, GV 20)

For screen growing in the eye: Liver *Shu* (*Gan Shu*, Bl 18), Life Gate (*Ming Men*, GV 4), Pupil Bone-Hole (*Tong Zi Liao*, GB 1) [5 *fen* lateral to the outer canthus; drain after qi is obtained], Union Valley (*He Gu*, LI 4), and Shang Yang (*Shang Yang*, LI 1)

For bird's eye in children (*i.e.,*) inability to see at night: Moxa 1 *cun* proximal to the nail of the thumb and the white flesh border at the end of the joint crease on the inner (*i.e.*, palmar) aspect of the thumb, each with 1 cone.

The Category of the Nose & Mouth

For polyps in the nose: Welcome Fragrance (*Ying Xiang*, LI 20)

For bleeding: Wind Mansion (*Feng Fu*, GV 16), Pool at the Bend (*Qu Chi*, LI 11), Union Valley (*He Gu*, LI 4), Third Space (*San Jian*, LI 3), Second Space (*Er Jian*, LI 2), Back Ravine (*Hou Xi*, SI 3), Front Valley (*Qian Gu*, SI 2), Bend Middle (*Wei Zhong*, Bl 40), Extending Vessel (*Shen Mai*, Bl 62), Kunlun (Mountain, *Kun Lun*, Bl 60), Severe Mouth (*Li Dui*, St 45), Upper Star (*Shang Xing*, GV 23), and Hidden White (*Yin Bai*, Sp 1)

For runny snivel nosebleed: Wind Mansion (*Feng Fu*, GV 16), Second Space (*Er Jian*, LI 2), and Welcome Fragrance (*Ying Xiang*, LI 20)

For nasal congestion: Upper Star (*Shang Xing*, GV 23), (Head) Overlooking Tears (*Lin Qi*, GB 15), Hundred Convergences (*Bai Hui*, GV 20), Front Valley (*Qian Gu*, SI 2), Severe Mouth (*Li Dui*, St 45), Union Valley (*He Gu*, LI 4), and Welcome Fragrance (*Ying Xiang*, LI 20)

For runny nose with clear nasal mucus: Human Center (*Ren Zhong*, GV 26), Upper Star (*Shang Xing*, GV 23), and Wind Mansion (*Feng Fu*, GV 16)

For brain abscess with foul mucus running from the nose: Deviating Turn (*Qu Cha*, Bl 4) and Upper Star (*Shang Xing*, GV 23)

For nosebleed: Upper Star (*Shang Xing*, GV 23) [moxa with 2 times 7 cones], Severed Bone (*Jue Gu*, GB 39), and Fontanel Meeting (*Xin Hui*, GV 22). Another method is to moxa at the depression between the two sinews at the hairline on the nape of the neck.

For enduring illness of uncheckable running of snivel: Hundred Convergences (*Bai Hui*, GV 20) [moxa]

For dry mouth: Cubit Marsh (*Chi Ze*, Lu 5), Marsh at the Bend (*Qu Ze*, Per 3), Great Mound (*Da Ling*, Per 7), Second Space (*Er Jian*, LI 2), Lesser Shang (*Shao Shang*, Lu 11), and Shang Yang (*Shang Yang*, LI 1)

For dry throat: Great Abyss (*Tai Yuan*, Lu 9) and Fish Border (*Yu Ji*, Lu 10)

For wasting thirst: Water Trough (*Shui Gou*, GV 26), Sauce Receptacle (*Cheng Jiang*, CV 24), Gold Liquid (*Jin Jing*, M-HN-20-b), Jade Humor (*Yu Ye*, M-HN-20a), Pool at the Bend (*Qu Chi*, LI 11), Palace of Toil (*Lao Gong*, Per 8), Supreme Surge (*Tai Chong*, Liv 3), Moving Between (*Xing Jian*, Liv 2), Shang Hill (*Shang Qiu*, Sp 5), Blazing Valley (*Ran Gu*, Ki 2), and Hidden White (*Yin Bai*, Sp 1). [Do not moxa by any means if the condition has lasted over 100 days.]

For dry lips with drooling: Lower Ridge (*Xia Lian*, LI 8)

For dry tongue with drooling: Recover Flow (*Fu Liu*, Ki 7)

For dry lips with no desire for drinks: Third Space (*San Jian*, LI 3) and Lesser Shang (*Shao Shang*, Lu 11)

For lips moving like worms wriggling: Water Trough (*Shui Gou*, GV 26)

For swollen lips: Welcome Fragrance (*Ying Xiang*, LI 20)

For deviated mouth and eyes: Jawbone (*Jia Che*, St 6), Water Trough (*Shui Gou*, GV 26), Broken Sequence (*Lie Que*, Lu 7), Great Abyss (*Tai Yuan*, Lu 9), Union Valley (*He Gu*, LI 4), Second Space (*Er Jian*, LI 2), Earth Granary (*Di Cang*, St 4), and Silk Bamboo Hole (*Si Zhu Kong*, TH 23)

For clenched jaw: Jawbone (*Jia Che*, St 6), Branch Ditch (*Zhi Gou*, TH 6), Outer Pass (*Wai Guan*, TH 5), Broken Sequence (*Lie Que*, Lu 7), Inner Court (*Nei Ting*, St 44), and Severe Mouth (*Li Dui*, St 45)

For loss of voice: Intermediary Courier (*Jian Shi*, Per 5), Branch Ditch (*Zhi Gou*, TH 6), Spirit Pathway (*Ling Dao*, Ht 4), Fish Border (*Yu Ji*, Lu 10), Union Valley (*He Gu*, LI 4), Yin Valley (*Yin Gu*, Ki 10), Recover Flow (*Fu Liu*, Ki 7), and Blazing Valley (*Ran Gu*, Ki 2)

For slack tongue: Great Abyss (*Tai Yuan*, Lu 9), Union Valley (*He Gu*, LI 4), Surging Yang (*Chong Yang*, St 42), Inner Court (*Nei Ting*, St 44), Kunlun (Mountain, *Kun Lun*, Bl 60), Three Yin Intersection (*San Yin Jiao*, Sp 6), and Wind Mansion (*Feng Fu*, GV 16)

For stiff tongue: Mute's Gate (*Ya Men*, GV 15), Lesser Shang (*Shao Shang*, Lu 11), Fish Border (*Yu Ji*, Lu 10), Second Space (*Er Jian*, LI 2), Central Hub (*Zhong Chong*, Per 9), Yin Valley (*Yin Gu*, Ki 10), and Blazing Valley (*Ran Gu*, Ki 2)

For yellowing of the tongue: Fish Border (*Yu Ji*, Lu 10)

For cold teeth: Lesser Sea (*Shao Hai*, Ht 3)

For toothache: Shang Yang (*Shang Yang*, LI 1)

For decayed teeth with aversion to wind: Union Valley (*He Gu*, LI 4) and Severe Mouth (*Li Dui*, St 45)

For tooth decay: Lesser Sea (*Shao Hai*, Ht 3), Small Sea (*Xiao Hai*, SI 8), Yang Valley (*Yang Gu*, SI 5), Union Valley (*He Gu*, LI 4), Humor Gate (*Ye Men*, TH 2), Second Space (*Er Jian*, LI 2), Inner Court (*Nei Ting*, St 44), and Severe Mouth (*Li Dui*, St 45)

For pain of the gums: Angle Vertex (*Jiao Sun*, TH 20) and Small Sea (*Xiao Hai*, SI 8)

For erosion of the tongue and teeth: Sauce Receptacle (*Cheng Jiang*, CV 24) and Palace of Toil (*Lao Gong*, Per 8) [each 1 cone]

For toothache: Pool at the Bend (*Qu Chi*, LI 11), Lesser Sea (*Shao Hai*, Ht 3), Yang Valley (*Yang Gu*, SI 5), Yang Ravine (*Yang Xi*, LI 5), Second Space (*Er Jian*, LI 2), Humor Gate (*Ye Men*, TH 2), Jawbone (*Jia Che*, St 6), Inner Court (*Nei Ting*, St 44), and Small Lu (*Lu Xi*, i.e., Great Ravine, *Tai Xi*, Ki 3) [at the top of the inner malleolus; moxa with 2 times 7 cones]

For upper toothache (*i.e.*, aching among the upper teeth): Human Center (*Ren Zhong*, GV 26), Great Abyss (*Tai Yuan*, Lu 9), and Small Lu (*Lu Xi*, i.e., Great Ravine, *Tai Xi*, Ki 3). (In addition,) moxa the prominent muscle in the upper arm with 5 cones.

For lower toothache: Dragon Black (*Long Xuan*) [at the crossed vessels on the lateral aspect of the wrist], Sauce Receptacle (*Cheng Jiang*, CV 24), and Union Valley (*He Gu*, LI 4). (In addition,) moxa 5 *cun* proximal to the wrist between the two sinews with 5 cones.

For inability to chew: Angle Vertex (*Jiao Sun*, TH 20)

For tooth *gan* with erosion and ulceration[1] and sores: Sauce Receptacle (*Cheng Jiang*, CV 24). [Moxa with 7 cones. The size of the cones should be the size of the small end of a chopstick.]

---

[1]   Tooth *gan* means swollen gums with ulceration.

The Category of Chest, Upper Back & Lateral Costal Regions

For chest fullness: Channel Ditch (*Jing Qu*, Lu 8), Yang Ravine (*Yang Xi*, LI 5), Back Ravine (*Hou Xi*, SI 3), Third Space (*San Jian*, LI 3), Intermediary Courier (*Jian Shi*, Per 5), Yang Mound (Spring) (*Yang Ling*, GB 34), (Leg) Three *Li* (*San Li*, St 36), Spring at the Bend (*Qu Quan*, Liv 8), and Foot Overlooking Tears (*Zu Lin Qi*, GB 41)

For chest *bi*[1]: Great Abyss (*Tai Yuan*, Lu 9)

For oppression in the chest and the upper arms: Shoulder Well (*Jian Jing*, GB 21)

For pain in the chest and flanks: Celestial Well (*Tian Jing*, TH 10), Branch Ditch (*Zhi Gou*, TH 6), Intermediary Courier (*Jian Shi*, Per 5), Great Mound (*Da Ling*, Per 7), (Arm) Three *Li* (*San Li*, LI 10)[2], Supreme White (*Tai Bai*, Sp 3), Hill Ruins (*Qiu Xu*, GB 40), and Yang Assistance (*Yang Fu*, GB 38)

For a rolling sensation in the chest: Intermediary Courier (*Jian Shi*, Per 5)

---

[1] Chest *bi* is chest pain due to block and oppression. Another definition says that it is chest fullness and oppression with pain arising upon eating food, inability to swallow food, and occasional retching.

[2] Leg Three *Li* (*Zu San Li*, St 36) may be meant here instead, or both Leg and Arm Three *Li*.

For fullness and propping up swelling of the chest: Inner Pass (*Nei Guan*, Per 6) and Diaphragm *Shu* (*Ge Shu*, Bl 17)

For chest and flank fullness giving a dragging sensation in the abdomen: Lower Ridge (*Xia Lian*, St 39), Hill Ruins (*Qiu Xu*, GB 40), Pinched Ravine (*Xia Xi*, GB 43), and Kidney *Shu* (*Shen Shu*, Bl 23)

For chest vexation: Cycle Gate (*Qi Men*, Liv 14)

For cold in the chest: Chest Center (*Dan Zhong*, CV 17)

For aching pain in the shoulder and upper back: Wind Gate (*Feng Men*, Bl 12), Shoulder Well (*Jian Jing*, GB 21), Central Islet (*Zhong Zhu*, TH 3), Branch Ditch (*Zhi Gou*, TH 6), Back Ravine (*Hou Xi*, SI 3), Wrist Bone (*Wan Gu*, SI 4), and Bend Middle (*Wei Zhong*, Bl 40)

For heart and chest pain: Marsh at the Bend (*Qu Ze*, Per 3), Inner Pass (*Nei Guan*, Per 6), and Great Mound (*Da Ling*, Per 7)

For fullness of the chest with blood inflation and accumulation lumps, sudden turmoil with rumbling intestines, and frequent belching: (Leg) Three *Li* (*San Li*, St 36) and Cycle Gate (*Qi Men*, Liv 14). [Needle 2 *cun* laterally with neither supplementation nor drainage.]

For fullness of the flanks: Screen Gate (*Zhang Men*, Liv 13)

For flank pain: Yang Valley (*Yang Gu*, SI 5), Wrist Bone (*Wan Gu*, SI 4), Branch Ditch (*Zhi Gou*, TH 6), Diaphragm *Shu* (*Ge Shu*, Bl 17), and Extending Vessel (*Shen Mai*, Bl 62)

For swelling of the supraclavicular fossa: Great Abyss (*Tai Yuan*, Lu 9), Shang Yang (*Shang Yang*, LI 1), and Foot Overlooking Tears (*Zu Lin Qi*, GB 41)

For mutual dragging between the flanks and the spine: Liver *Shu* (*Gan Shu*, Bl 18)

For hypertonicity of the upper back, upper arms, and nape of the neck: Great Vertebra (*Da Zhui*, GV 14)

For rigidity of the upper and lower back with inability to turn about: Lumbar *Shu* (*Yao Shu*, GV 2) and Lung *Shu* (*Fei Shu*, Bl 13)

For pain and discomfort of the lumbar spine: Bend Middle (*Wei Zhong*, Bl 40) and Recover Flow (*Fu Liu*, Ki 7)

For stooped upper and lower back: Wind Pool (*Feng Chi*, GB 20) and Lung *Shu* (*Fei Shu*, Bl 13)

For hypertonicity of the back: Channel Ditch (*Jing Qu*, Lu 8)

For mutual dragging between the shoulders and the back: Second Space (*Er Jian*, LI 2), Shang Yang (*Shang Yang*, LI 1), Bend Middle (*Wei Zhong*, Bl 40), and Kunlun (Mountain, *Kun Lun*, Bl 60)

For hemilateral painful *bi* of the flank and back: Fish Border (*Yu Ji*, Lu 10) and Bend Middle (*Wei Zhong*, Bl 40)

For backache: Channel Ditch (*Jing Qu*, Lu 8), Hill Ruins (*Qiu Xu*, GB 40), Fish Border (*Yu Ji*, Lu 10), Kunlun (Mountain, *Kun Lun*, Bl 60), and Capital Bone (*Jing Gu*, Bl 64)

For stiffness and pain of the spine and paravertebral sinews: Bend Middle (*Wei Zhong*, Bl 40)

For a dragging pain in and difficulty turning about the upper and lower back: Celestial Window (*Tian You*, TH 16), Wind Pool

(*Feng Chi*, GB 20), Union Valley (*He Gu*, LI 4), and Kunlun (Mountain, *Kun Lun*, Bl 60)

For a dragging pain inside the spine with inability either to bend or to stretch (the back): Union Valley (*He Gu*, LI 4), Recover Flow (*Fu Liu*, Ki 7), and Kunlun (Mountain, *Kun Lun*, Bl 60)

For stiffness of the spine with pain all over the body and inability to turn about: Mute's Gate (*Ya Men*, GV 15)

For chest pain radiating to the flanks: Cycle Gate (*Qi Men*, Liv 14) [needle first], Screen Gate (*Zhang Men*, Liv 13), Hill Ruins (*Qiu Xu*, GB 40), Moving Between (*Xing Jian*, Liv 2), and Gushing Spring (*Yong Quan*, Ki 1)

For *bi* pain in the shoulder: Shoulder Bone (*Jian Yu*, LI 15), Celestial Well (*Tian Jing*, TH 10), Pool at the Bend (*Qu Chi*, LI 11), Yang Valley (*Yang Gu*, SI 5), and Passage Hub (*Guan Chong*, TH 1)

The Category of the Hands, Feet, Lumbus & Axillae

For pain in and inability to lift the hand and arm: Pool at the Bend (*Qu Chi*, LI 11), Cubit Marsh (*Chi Ze*, Lu 5), Shoulder Bone (*Jian Yu*, LI 15), (Arm) Three *Li* (*San Li*, LI 10), Lesser Sea (*Shao Hai*, Ht 3), Great Abyss (*Tai Yuan*, Lu 9), Yang Pool (*Yang Chi*, TH 4), Yang Ravine (*Yang Xi*, LI 5), Yang Valley (*Yang Gu*, SI 5), Front Valley (*Qian Gu*, SI 2), Union Valley (*He Gu*, LI 4), Humor Gate (*Ye Men*, TH 2), Outer Pass (*Wai Guan*, TH 5), and Wrist Bone (*Wan Gu*, SI 4)

For cold arm: Cubit Marsh (*Chi Ze*, Lu 5) and Spirit Gate (*Shen Men*, Ht 7)

For pain in the inner aspect of the arm: Great Abyss (*Tai Yuan*, Lu 9)

For pain in the lateral aspect of arm and wrist: Yang Valley (*Yang Gu*, SI 5)

For trembling and rocking of the hand and wrist: Marsh at the Bend (*Qu Ze*, Per 3)

For pain in the armpit: Lesser Sea (*Shao Hai*, Ht 3), Intermediary Courier (*Jian Shi*, Per 5), Lesser Mansion (*Shao Fu*, Ht 8), Yang Assistance (*Yang Fu*, GB 38), Hill Ruins (*Qiu Xu*, GB 40), Foot Overlooking Tears (*Zu Lin Qi*, GB 41), and Extending Vessel (*Shen Mai*, Bl 62)

For elbow taxation[1]: Celestial Well (*Tian Jing*, TH 10), Pool at the Bend (*Qu Chi*, LI 11), Intermediary Courier (*Jian Shi*, Per 5), Yang Ravine (*Yang Xi*, LI 5), Central Islet (*Zhong Zhu*, TH 3), Yang Valley (*Yang Gu*, SI 5), Great Abyss (*Tai Yuan*, Lu 9), Wrist Bone (*Wan Gu*, SI 4), Broken Sequence (*Lie Que*, Lu 7), and Humor Gate (*Ye Men*, TH 2)

For flaccid hand and wrist: Broken Sequence (*Lie Que*, Lu 7)

For pain in the elbow and arm: Shoulder Bone (*Jian Yu*, LI 15), Pool at the Bend (*Qu Chi*, LI 11), Connecting the Interior (*Tong Li*, Ht 5), and Arm Three Li (*Shou San Li*, LI 10)

For hypertonicity of the elbow: Cubit Marsh (*Chi Ze*, Lu 5), Shoulder Bone (*Jian Yu*, LI 15), Small Sea (*Xiao Hai*, SI 8), Intermediary Courier (*Jian Shi*, Per 5), Great Mound (*Da Ling*, Per 7), Back Ravine (*Hou Xi*, SI 3), and Fish Border (*Yu Ji*, Lu 10)

For aching and heaviness of the shoulder and arm: Branch Ditch (*Zhi Gou*, TH 6)

For inability to contract the elbow, arm, and fingers: Pool at the Bend (*Qu Chi*, LI 11), (Arm) Three Li (*San Li*, LI 10), Outer Pass (*Wai Guan*, TH 5), and Central Islet (*Zhong Zhu*, TH 3)

For numbness and insensitivity of the hand and arm: Celestial Well (*Tian Jing*, TH 10), Pool at the Bend (*Qu Chi*, LI 11), Outer Pass (*Wai Guan*, TH 5), Channel Ditch (*Jing Qu*, Lu 8), Branch Ditch (*Zhi Gou*, TH 6), Yang Ravine (*Yang Xi*, LI 5), Wrist Bone (*Wan Gu*, SI 4), Upper Ridge (*Shang Lian*, LI 9), and Union Valley (*He Gu*, LI 4)

---

[1] Elbow taxation refers to a disabled elbow due to straining, overwork, or contraction of wind cold.

For cold and pain in the hand and arm: Shoulder Well (*Jian Jing*, GB 21), Pool at the Bend (*Qu Chi*, LI 11), and Lower Ridge (*Xia Lian*, LI 8)

For hypertonicity of the fingers with the sinews stiff (*i.e.*, tense): Pool at the Bend (*Qu Chi*, LI 11), Yang Valley (*Yang Gu*, SI 5), and Union Valley (*He Gu*, LI 4)

For hotness in the hand: Palace of Toil (*Lao Gong*, Per 8), Pool at the Bend (*Qu Chi*, LI 11), Marsh at the Bend (*Qu Ze*, Per 3), Inner Pass (*Nei Guan*, Per 6), Broken Sequence (*Lie Que*, Lu 7), Channel Ditch (*Jing Qu*, Lu 8), Great Abyss (*Tai Yuan*, Lu 9), Central Hub (*Zhong Chong*, Per 9), and Lesser Surge (*Shao Chong*, Ht 9)

For redness and swelling of the hand and arm: Pool at the Bend (*Qu Chi*, LI 11), Connecting the Interior (*Tong Li*, Ht 5), Central Islet (*Zhong Zhu*, TH 3), Union Valley (*He Gu*, LI 4), Arm Three Li (*Shou San Li*, LI 10), and Humor Gate (*Ye Men*, TH 2)

For wind *bi* with hypertonicity of and inability to lift the arm: Cubit Marsh (*Chi Ze*, Lu 5), Pool at the Bend (*Qu Chi*, LI 11), and Union Valley (*He Gu*, LI 4)

For hypertonicity of the hand, hemilateral wind, erratic papules[2], throat *bi*, stuffy fullness of the chest and flanks, slack sinews with flaccidity of the hand and arm, and withered, parched skin: Pool at the Bend (*Qu Chi*, LI 11) [first drain, then supplement], Shoulder Bone (*Jian Yu*, LI 15) and Arm Three Li (*Shou San Li*, LI 10)

---

[2] Erratic papules mean urticaria or dormant papule according to Wiseman *et al*. They are so named because they recur unpredictably.

For distressed aching of the shoulder and upper arm: Shoulder Bone (*Jian Yu*, LI 15), Shoulder Well (*Jian Jing*, GB 21), and Pool at the Bend (*Qu Chi*, LI 11)

For aching all over the five fingers: Outer Pass (*Wai Guan*, TH 5)

For hypertonicity of the hand with pain in the fingers: Lesser Shang (*Shao Shang*, Lu 11)

For hotness in the palms: Broken Sequence (*Lie Que*, Lu 7), Channel Ditch (*Jing Qu*, Lu 8), and Great Abyss (*Tai Yuan*, Lu 9)

For swelling of the armpit and elbow: Cubit Marsh (*Chi Ze*, Lu 5), Small Sea (*Xiao Hai*, SI 8), Intermediary Courier (*Jian Shi*, Per 5), and Great Mound (*Da Ling*, Per 7)

For swelling under the armpit: Yang Assistance (*Yang Fu*, GB 38), Hill Ruins (*Qiu Xu*, GB 40), and Foot Overlooking Tears (*Zu Lin Qi*, GB 41)

For low back pain: Shoulder Well (*Jian Jing*, GB 21), Jumping Round (*Huan Tiao*, GB 30), Yin Market (*Yin Shi*, St 33), (Leg) Three *Li* (*San Li*, St 36), Bend Middle (*Wei Zhong*, Bl 40), Mountain Support (*Cheng Shan*, Bl 57), Yang Assistance (*Yang Fu*, GB 38), Kunlun (Mountain, *Kun Lun*, Bl 60), Lumbar *Shu* (*Yao Shu*, GV 2), and Kidney *Shu* (*Shen Shu*, Bl 23)

For ice-cold of the legs: Yin Market (*Yin Shi*, St 33)

For low back pain due to wrenching and contusion and pain in the region of the free ribs: Cubit Marsh (*Chi Ze*, Lu 5), Pool at the Bend (*Qu Chi*, LI 11), Union Valley (*He Gu*, LI 4), Arm Three *Li* (*Shou San Li*, LI 10), Yin Mound (Spring) (*Yin Ling*, Sp 9), Yin Intersection (*Yin Jiao*, CV 7), Moving Between (*Xing Jian*, Liv 2), and Leg Three *Li* (*Zu San Li*, St 36)

For pain in and difficulty moving the lumbus: Wind Market (*Feng Shi*, GB 31), Bend Middle (*Wei Zhong*, Bl 40), and Moving Between (*Xing Jian*, Liv 2)

For stiffness and pain of the lumbar spine: Lumbar *Shu* (*Yao Shu*, GV 2), Bend Middle (*Wei Zhong*, Bl 40), Gushing Spring (*Yong Quan*, Ki 1), Small Intestine *Shu* (*Xiao Chang Shu*, Bl 27), and Bladder *Shu* (*Pang Guang Shu*, Bl 28)

For pain in the lumbus and feet: Jumping Round (*Huan Tiao*, GB 30), Wind Market (*Feng Shi*, GB 31), Yin Market (*Yin Shi*, St 33), Bend Middle (*Wei Zhong*, Bl 40), Mountain Support (*Cheng Shan*, Bl 57), Kunlun (Mountain, *Kun Lun*, Bl 60), and Extending Vessel (*Shen Mai*, Bl 62)

For pain inside the thigh and knee: Bend Middle (*Wei Zhong*, Bl 40), (Leg) Three *Li* (*San Li*, St 36), and Three Yin Intersection (*San Yin Jiao*, Sp 6)

For aching pain in the leg and knee: Jumping Round (*Huan Tiao*, GB 30), Yang Mound (Spring) (*Yang Ling*, GB 34), and Hill Ruins (*Qiu Xu*, GB 40)

For pain in the foot and knee: Bend Middle (*Wei Zhong*, Bl 40), (Leg) Three *Li* (*San Li*, St 36), Spring at the Bend (*Qu Quan*, Liv 8), Yang Mound (Spring) (*Yang Ling*, GB 34), Wind Market (*Feng Shi*, GB 31), Kunlun (Mountain, *Kun Lun*, Bl 60), and Ravine Divide (*Jie Xi*, St 41)

For swelling in the knee, lower leg, and thigh: Bend Middle (*Wei Zhong*, Bl 40), (Leg) Three *Li* (*San Li*, St 36), Yang Assistance (*Yang Fu*, GB 38), Ravine Divide (*Jie Xi*, St 41), and Mountain Support (*Cheng Shan*, Bl 57)

For the lumbus (cold) as if sitting in water: Yang Assistance (*Yang Fu*, GB 38)

For atonic foot with inability to move: Recover Flow (*Fu Liu*, Ki 7)

For wind *bi* with numbness and insensitivity of the foot and lower leg: Jumping Round (*Huan Tiao*, GB 30) and Wind Market (*Feng Shi*, GB 31)

For *bi* numbness of the foot: Jumping Round (*Huan Tiao*, GB 30), Yin Mound (Spring) (*Yin Ling*, Sp 9), Yang Mound (Spring) (*Yang Ling*, GB 34), Yang Assistance (*Yang Fu*, GB 38), Great Ravine (*Tai Xi*, Ki 3), and Reaching Yin (*Zhi Yin*, Bl 67)

For foot qi[3]: Shoulder Well (*Jian Jing*, GB 21), Eye of the Knee (*Xi Yan*, M-LE-16a), Wind Market (*Feng Shi*, GB 31), (Leg) Three *Li* (*San Li*, St 36), Mountain Support (*Cheng Shan*, Bl 57), Supreme Surge (*Tai Chong*, Liv 3), Hill Ruins (*Qiu Xu*, GB 40), and Moving Between (*Xing Jian*, Liv 2)

For pain in the acetabular region: Jumping Round (*Huan Tiao*, GB 30), Yang Mound (Spring) (*Yang Ling*, GB 34), and Hill Ruins (*Qiu Xu*, GB 40)

For cold and heat of the foot: (Leg) Three *Li* (*San Li*, St 36), Bend Middle (*Wei Zhong*, Bl 40), Yang Mound (Spring) (*Yang Ling*, GB 34), Recover Flow (*Fu Liu*, Ki 7), Blazing Valley (*Ran Gu*, Ki 2), Moving Between (*Xing Jian*, Liv 2), Mound Center (*Zhong Feng*, Liv 4), Great Metropolis (*Da Du*, Sp 2), and Hidden White (*Yin Bai*, Sp 1)

For swollen foot: Mountain Support (*Cheng Shan*, Bl 57), Kunlun (Mountain, *Kun Lun*, Bl 60), Blazing Valley (*Ran Gu*, Ki 2), Bend

---

[3] Foot qi refers to swelling starting from the feet usually accompanied by numbness and insensitivity. It may progress upward toward the heart to cause a series of heart problems.

Middle (*Wei Zhong*, Bl 40), Lower Ridge (*Xia Lian*, St 39), Hip Bone (*Kuan Gu*, GB 30), and Wind Market (*Feng Shi*, GB 31)

For ice cold of the foot: Kidney *Shu* (*Shen Shu*, Bl 23)

For shivering of the whole body and aching of the lower leg: Mountain Support (*Cheng Shan*, Bl 57) and Metal Gate (*Jin Men*, Bl 63)

For cold of the foot and lower leg: Recover Flow (*Fu Liu*, Ki 7), Extending Vessel (*Shen Mai*, Bl 62), and Severe Mouth (*Li Dui*, St 45)

For hypertonicity of the foot: Kidney *Shu* (*Shen Shu*, Bl 23), Yang Mound (Spring) (*Yang Ling*, GB 34), Yang Assistance (*Yang Fu*, GB 38), and Severed Bone (*Jue Gu*, GB 39)

For pain in all the joints (of the body): Yang Assistance (*Yang Fu*, GB 38)

For swelling of the calf: Mountain Support (*Cheng Shan*, Bl 57) and Kunlun (Mountain, *Kun Lun*, Bl 60)

For slack feet: Yang Mound (Spring) (*Yang Ling*, GB 34), Surging Yang (*Chong Yang*, St 42), Supreme Surge (*Tai Chong*, Liv 3), and Hill Ruins (*Qiu Xu*, GB 40)

For weakness of the feet: Bend Middle (*Wei Zhong*, Bl 40), (Leg) Three *Li* (*San Li*, St 36), and Mountain Support (*Cheng Shan*, Bl 57)

For redness, swelling, aching, and pain of the knee: Knee Joint (*Xi Guan*, Liv 7), Bend Middle (*Wei Zhong*, Bl 40), (Leg) Three *Li* (*San Li*, St 36), and Yin Market (*Yin Shi*, St 33)

For heel-penetrating straw-sandal wind[4]: Kunlun (Mountain, *Kun Lun*, Bl 60), Hill Ruins (*Qiu Xu*, GB 40), Shang Hill (*Shang Qiu*, Sp 5), and Shining Sea (*Zhao Hai*, Ki 6)

For the feet being unable to walk: (Leg) Three *Li* (*San Li*, St 36), Spring at the Bend (*Qu Quan*, Liv 8), Bend Middle (*Wei Zhong*, Bl 40), Yang Assistance (*Yang Fu*, GB 38), Three Yin Intersection (*San Yin Jiao*, Sp 6), Recover Flow (*Fu Liu*, Ki 7), Surging Yang (*Chong Yang*, St 42), Blazing Valley (*Ran Gu*, Ki 2), Extending Vessel (*Shen Mai*, Bl 62), Moving Between (*Xing Jian*, Liv 2), and Spleen *Shu* (*Pi Shu*, Bl 20)

For aching of the ankle: Bend Middle (*Wei Zhong*, Bl 40) and Kunlun (Mountain, *Kun Lun*, Bl 60)

For pain in the center of the foot (*i.e.*, the center of the sole): Kunlun (Mountain, *Kun Lun*, Bl 60)

For shortened (*i.e.*, contracted) and tense foot sinews, heaviness of the feet, crane's knee wind[5], and articular wind swelling[6] with aversion to wind and inability to rise up during the attack: Wind Market (*Feng Shi*, GB 31)

---

[4] Straw-sandal wind is a problem ascribed to the kidneys. It is manifested by skin lesions, usually pox starting from the heels and hips, which, whether itching or not, may break open giving rise to sores, swelling, or scarring and which may extend to the soles.

[5] Crane's knee wind refers to swollen knee joints with thin lower legs due to long-lasting *bi* which is, in turn, caused by invasion of wind cold.

[6] Articular wind is caused by the evil qi of wind and dampness. It manifests as red swelling and restriction of the mobility of the joints which may be very painful. In severe cases, it may be accompanied by fever, shortness of breath, spontaneous sweating, dizziness, desire to vomit, etc.

For low back pain with inability to stand for long, aching and heaviness of the leg, knee, and tibia, and inability to lift the limbs: Instep Yang (*Fu Yang*, Bl 59)

For heaviness of and unbearable pain in the lumbus with difficulty in turning over, rising up, and lying down, frigidity *bi*[7], and hypertonicity of and inability to stretch or contract the feet sinews: Moxa the ends of the creases of the popliteal fossae, four points altogether, each with 3 cones. Moxa them simultaneously, (the cones) being blown at the same time by two persons at either side till the fires die out. If moxibustion is performed at noon and toward evening there appears rumbling in the viscera and bowels or there are one or two bowel movements, the illness will be cured thereupon.

For pain in and inability to lift (*i.e.*, move) the lumbus: Servant Kneeling (*Pu Can*, Bl 61) [Two points, located in the depressions under the heelbones. Locate them with the foot arched. Moxa with 2 cones.]

For illnesses above the knee: Moxa Jumping Round (*Huan Tiao*, GB 30) and Wind Market (*Feng Shi*, GB 31).

For illnesses below the knee: Moxa Calf's Nose (*Du Bi*, St 35), Knee Joint (*Xi Guan*, Liv 7), (Leg) Three *Li* (*San Li*, St 36), and Yang Mound (Spring) (*Yang Ling*, GB 34).

For illnesses above the ankle: Moxa Three Yin Intersection (*San Yin Jiao*, Sp 6), Severed Bone (*Jue Gu*, GB 39), and Kunlun (Mountain, *Kun Lun*, Bl 60).

---

7   Frigidity *bi* is cold *bi* whose signs and symptoms include agonizing pain of the limb joints exacerbated by exposure to cold but relieved on exposure to warmth.

For illnesses below the ankle: Moxa Shining Sea (*Zhao Hai*, Ki 6) and Extending Vessel (*Shen Mai*, Bl 62).

For pain in the leg: Hip Bone (*Kuan Gu*, GB 30)

For foot qi: First, Wind Market (*Feng Shi*, GB 31) [100 or 50 cones]; second, Crouching Rabbit (*Fu Tu*, St 32) [needled 3 *fen* deep; moxa prohibited]; third, Calf's Nose (*Du Bi*, St 35) [50 cones]; fourth, Eye of the Knee (*Xi Yan*, M-LE-16a); fifth, (Leg) Three *Li* (*San Li*, St 36) [100 cones]; sixth, Upper Ridge (*Shang Lian*, St 37); seventh, Lower Ridge (*Xia Lian*, St 37) [100 cones]; eighth, Severed Bone (*Jue Gu*, GB 39)

For cramps of the feet which become unendurable during the attack: The top of the malleolus [1 cone]. Moxa the inner in case of cramps on the medial side, and moxa the outer in case of cramps on the lateral side.

For cramps of the feet which have persisted for years and for which all the various formulas have proven ineffective: Moxa Mountain Support (*Cheng Shan*, Bl 57) [2 times 7 cones].

The Category of Women

For menstrual irregularity: Sea of Qi (*Qi Hai*, CV 6), Central Pole (*Zhong Ji*, CV 3), Girdling Vessel (*Dai Mai*, GB 26) [1 cone], Kidney *Shu* (*Shen Shu*, Bl 23), and Three Yin Intersection (*San Yin Jiao*, Sp 6)

For inhibited menstrual flow[1]: Foot Overlooking Tears (*Zu Lin Qi*, GB 41), Three Yin Intersection (*San Yin Jiao*, Sp 6), and Central Pole (*Zhong Ji*, CV 3)

For menstrual flow persisting beyond due course: Hidden White (*Yin Bai*, Sp 1)

For menstrual flow accompanied by (generalized) cold and coming on at no regular intervals: Origin Pass (*Guan Yuan*, CV 4)

For incessant dribbling uterine bleeding in women: Supreme Surge (*Tai Chong*, Liv 3) and Three Yin Intersection (*San Yin Jiao*, Sp 6)

For profuse uterine bleeding: Sea of Qi (*Qi Hai*, CV 6), Great Pile (*Da Dun*, Liv 1), Yin Valley (*Yin Gu*, Ki 10), Supreme Surge (*Tai Chong*, Liv 3), Blazing Valley (*Ran Gu*, Ki 2), Three Yin Intersection (*San Yin Jiao*, Sp 6), and Central Pole (*Zhong Ji*, CV 3)

---

[1] Inhibited menstrual flow means obstructed menstruation accompanied by lower abdominal pain.

For conglomeration and gathering: Origin Pass (*Guan Yuan*, CV 4)

For red and white vaginal discharge: Girdling Vessel (*Dai Mai*, GB 26), Origin Pass (*Guan Yuan*, CV 4), Sea of Qi (*Qi Hai*, CV 6), Three Yin Intersection (*San Yin Jiao*, Sp 6), White Ring *Shu* (*Bai Huan Shu*, Bl 30), and Intermediary Courier (*Jian Shi*, Per 5) [30 cones]

For hardness in the lower abdomen: Girdling Vessel (*Dai Mai*, GB 26)

For infertility: Shang Hill (*Shang Qiu*, Sp 5) and Central Pole (*Zhong Ji*, CV 3)

For persistent flow of lochia postpartum: Sea of Qi (*Qi Hai*, CV 6) and Origin Pass (*Guan Yuan*, CV 4)

For various diseases postpartum: Cycle Gate (*Qi Men*, Liv 14)

For mammary *yong*[2]: Lower Ridge (*Xia Lian*, St 39), (Leg) Three Li (*San Li*, St 36), Pinched Ravine (*Xia Xi*, GB 43), Fish Border (*Yu Ji*, Lu 10), Bend Middle (*Wei Zhong*, Bl 40), Foot Overlooking Tears (*Zu Lin Qi*, GB 41), and Lesser Marsh (*Shao Ze*, SI 1)

For mammary *yong* pain: Foot Overlooking Tears (*Zu Lin Qi*, GB 41)

For difficult delivery: Union Valley (*He Gu*, LI 4) [supplement], Three Yin Intersection (*San Yin Jiao*, Sp 6) [drain], and Supreme Surge (*Tai Chong*, Liv 3)

---

[2] Mammary *yong* is an acute inflammation of the breast which may be caused by a number of factors.

For death in utero due to transverse birth (*i.e.*, breech presentation): Supreme Surge (*Tai Chong*, Liv 3), Union Valley (*He Gu*, LI 4), and Three Yin Intersection (*San Yin Jiao*, Sp 6)

For transverse birth with hands coming out first: Tip of the small toe of the right foot. [Moxa with 3 cones and the child will be delivered thereupon. The cones should be the size of grains of wheat.]

For upsurge of the fetus pressing the heart[3] with qi oppression and bordering on expiry: Great Tower Gate (*Ju Que*, CV 14) and Union Valley (*He Gu*, LI 4) [supplement] and Three Yin Intersection (*San Yin Jiao*, Sp 6) [drain]. (While being needled,) the mother will feel her heart as if held by the child's hands. After birth, in the center of the palm, the left of a boy baby but the right of a girl baby, there is a mark to prove the needling. Otherwise, there will be a mark from needling on the philtrum or on the back of the head.

For postpartum blood dizziness with loss of consciousness of people: Branch Ditch (*Zhi Gou*, TH 6), (Leg) Three *Li* (*San Li*, St 36), and Three Yin Intersection (*San Yin Jiao*, Sp 6)

For ice-cold of the extremities and counterflow inversion (of the limbs) following abortion: Shoulder Well (*Jian Jing*, GB 21) [5 *fen* deep. In case oppression and distress is felt, supplement (Leg) Three *Li* {*San Li*, St 36} promptly.]

For retention of the placenta: Central Pole (*Zhong Ji*, CV 3) and Shoulder Well (*Jian Jing*, GB 21)

---

3   This is a sensation in the pregnant woman of something surging against her heart, often with fullness in the chest, which is due to counterflow of fetal qi.

For vaginal protrusion: Spring at the Bend (*Qu Quan*, Liv 8), Shining Sea (*Zhao Hai*, Ki 6), and Great Pile (*Da Dun*, Liv 1)

For absence of breast milk: Chest Center (*Dan Zhong*, CV 17) [moxa] and Lesser Marsh (*Shao Ze*, SI 1) [supplement]. These two points are divinely efficacious.

For blood clots: Spring at the Bend (*Qu Quan*, Liv 8), Recover Flow (*Fu Liu*, Ki 7), (Leg) Three *Li* (*San Li*, St 36), Sea of Qi (*Qi Hai*, CV 6), Cinnabar Field (*Dan Tian*, CV 5)[4], and Three Yin Intersection (*San Yin Jiao*, Sp 6)

For increasing emaciation, alternating cold and heat, and conflict between essence and blood in women due to intercourse with a man in the course of menstruation: Hundred Taxations (*Bai Lao*, i.e., Great Hammer, *Da Zhui*, GV 14), Kidney *Shu* (*Shen Shu*, Bl 23), Wind Gate (*Feng Men*, Bl 12), Central Pole (*Zhong Ji*, CV 3), Sea of Qi (*Qi Hai*, CV 6), and Three Yin Intersection (*San Yin Jiao*, Sp 6). It is wrong to treat this pattern as vacuity taxation.

For absence of menses in a woman with a yellow face, dry retching, but pregnancy not established: Pool at the Bend (*Qu Chi*, LI 11), Branch Ditch (*Zhi Gou*, TH 6), (Leg) Three *Li* (*San Li*, St 36), and Three Yin Intersection (*San Yin Jiao*, Sp 6)

For excessive channel vessels[5]: Connecting the Interior (*Tong Li*, Ht 5), Moving Between (*Xing Jian*, Liv 2), and Three Yin Intersection (*San Yin Jiao*, Sp 6)

---

[4] Because Origin Pass (*Guan Yuan*, CV 4) and Yin Intersection (*Yin Jiao*, CV 7) can also be called Cinnabar Field (*Dan Tian*) and are effective against similar disorders, either of these might possibly be meant instead.

[5] The translator suspects that excessive menstrual flow should be read for excessive channel vessels.

For desire to discontinue pregnancy: Moxa 1 *cun* above the medial malleolus of the right foot and Union Valley (*He Gu*, LI 4). Another method is to moxa 2 *cun* 3 *fen* below the navel with 3 cones and Shoulder Well (*Jian Jing*, GB 21).

For any types of cold exhaustion[6]: Moxa Origin Pass (*Guan Yuan*, CV 4).

For intermittent dribbling vaginal discharge: Three Yin Intersection (*San Yin Jiao*, Sp 6)

For menstrual irregularity and (blood) clots as a result of bind: Needle Intermediary Courier (*Jian Shi*, Per 5).

---

[6]   Cold exhaustion refers to a cold body and easy fatigue.

The Category of Children

For the five minor and major types of epilepsy[1]: Water Trough (*Shui Gou*, GV 26), Hundred Convergences (*Bai Hui*, GV 20), Spirit Gate (*Shen Men*, Ht 7), Metal Gate (*Jin Men*, Bl 63), Kunlun (Mountain, *Kun Lun*, Bl 60), and Great Tower Gate (*Ju Que*, CV 14)

For fright wind[2]: Wrist Bone (*Wan Gu*, SI 4)

For tugging and slackening and contracture of the five fingers: Yang Valley (*Yang Gu*, SI 5), Wrist Bone (*Wan Gu*, SI 4), and Kunlun (Mountain, *Kun Lun*, Bl 60)

For rocking of the head with the mouth open and arch-backed rigidity: Metal Gate (*Jin Men*, Bl 63)

For wind epilepsy[3] with upturned eyes: Hundred Convergences (*Bai Hui*, GV 20), Kunlun (Mountain, *Kun Lun*, Bl 60), and Silk Bamboo Hole (*Si Zhu Kong*, TH 23)

---

[1] The five epilepsies are horse-like, goat-like, chicken-like, swine-like, and cow-like epilepsy. Each is so named because the cry or groan of the patient is similar to the sound of the associated animal.

[2] Fright wind is of two types, acute and chronic. Its main manifestations are tugging and slackening, inversion, and clouded spirit.

[3] The signs and symptoms of wind epilepsy include dilated pupils, tremors of the limbs, shouting in dream, body heat, tugging and slackening, clenched jaw, rocking of the head, foaming at the mouth, and loss of consciousness. Its disease mechanism consists of insufficient heart qi and accumulated heat in the chest and provocation by intrusion of wind.

For prolapse of the rectum: Hundred Convergences (*Bai Hui*, GV 20) and Long Strong (*Chang Qiang*, GV 1)

For sudden *shan*: Supreme Surge (*Tai Chong*, Liv 3)

For arch-backed rigidity: Hundred Convergences (*Bai Hui*, GV 20)

For diarrhea and dysentery: Spirit Gate (*Shen Que*, CV 8)

For red migratory wind[4]: Hundred Convergences (*Bai Hui*, GV 20) and Bend Middle (*Wei Zhong*, Bl 40)

For cold dysentery in late autumn: Moxa on the pulsating vessels 2 and 3 *cun* under the navel.

For vomiting of milk: Moxa Center Palace (*Zhong Ting*, CV 16) [1 *cun* 6 *fen* under Chest Center {*Dan Zhong*, CV 17}].

For sudden epilepsy and swine-like epilepsy: Great Tower Gate (*Ju Que*, CV 14) [moxa with 3 cones]

For the mouth sore of ulcerated gums with strong, repulsive, foul smell: Moxa the two points of Palace of Toil (*Lao Gong*, Per 8), each with 1 cone.

For sudden infliction of abdominal pain with blackish, green-blue abdominal skin: Moxa the four (corners) one half *cun* lateral

---

[4] Red migratory wind commonly refers to a special category of cinnabar toxins of migratory nature. However, in infants and especially newborns, it refers to nothing but cinnabar toxins. Cinnabar toxins are characterized by bright red, local skin lesions which cause burning heat, pain, and swelling and which extend quickly in every direction.

(and above and below) the navel (each) with 3 cones and at one *cun* beneath the xiphoid process with 3 cones.

For fright epilepsy: [Moxa with 3 cones] the vertex on the top of the head and [moxa with 3 cones the size of a grain of wheat] the green-blue vessels behind the ears.

For wind epilepsy with the fingers contracted as if counting things: Moxa the depression in the hairline above the nose with 3 cones.

For red canthi (in children) aged 2-3 years: Moxa at 1 *cun* 5 *fen* proximal to and between the thumb and its next finger (possibly a little proximal to Union Valley, {*He Gu*, LI 4}; tr.) with 3 cones.

For nonclosure of the fontanel: 5 *fen* above and below the navel, two points. (Moxa) each with 3 cones. Before the moxa sores arise, the fontanel will already be closed.

For night crying: Moxa Hundred Convergences (*Bai Hui*, GV 20) with 3 cones.

For distention and sagging of one (external) kidney (*i.e.*, testicle): Origin Pass (*Guan Yuan*, CV 4). [Moxa with 3 times 7 cones, and Great Pile {*Da Dun*, Liv 1}, 7 cones.]

For deathlike swine(-like) epilepsy with foaming at the mouth: Great Tower Gate (*Jue Que*, CV 14) [3 cones]

For food epilepsy[5] which attacks following cold and heat and shivering as after a soaking: 5 *fen* above the xiphoid process, (moxa) with 3 cones.

---

[5] Food epilepsy is caused by irregularities in breastfeeding, *i.e.*, overfeeding.

For goat(-like) epilepsy: The joint under the ninth (thoracic) vertebra, [moxa with 3 cones]. Another method is (to moxa) Great Vertebra (*Da Zhui*, GV 14) with 3 cones.

For cow(-like) epilepsy: Turtledove Tail (*Jiu Wei*, CV 15) [3 cones]. Another method is (to moxa) Turtledove Tail (*Jiu Wei*, CV 15) and Great Vertebra (*Da Zhui*, GV 14) each with 3 cones.

For horse(-like) epilepsy: Servant Kneeling (*Pu Can*, Bl 61) [two points, each with 3 cones]. Another method is (to moxa) Wind Mansion (*Feng Fu*, GV 16) and Center of the Navel (*Qi Zhong*, *i.e.*, Spirit Gate, *Shen Que*, CV 8) each with 3 cones.

For dog(-like) epilepsy: The centers of the two palms, the foot *tai yang* (channel) and Rib Door (*Lei Hu*, possibly *Ben Shen*, GB 13) [Moxa each with 1 cone.]

For chicken(-like) epilepsy: The various foot channels[6] [each with 3 cones]

For tooth *gan*[7] with ulceration and decay: Sauce Receptacle (*Cheng Jiang*, CV 24). [It is alright either to needle or moxa it.]

---

[6] Because of the ambiguity of the Chinese, this may refer to the various *yang* channels at the feet.

[7] Tooth *gan* refers to swelling and ulceration of gums.

The Category of Sore Toxins

T o treat the sore toxins of *yong* and *ju*[1], perform the bamboo horse-riding moxa method. Use a thin bamboo stick to measure the arm of the patient, with one end fixed at Cubit Marsh (*Chi Ze*, Lu 5) on the crease (of the elbow). Align the stick along the flesh (of the forearm) and cut it off at the tip of the middle finger. Further, obtain a bamboo pole whose ends are set on two stools. Make the patient disrobe and ride on the pole with their feet barely touching the ground. Place the measured bamboo stick vertically on the pole along the back of the patient. Mark in ink the point (on the back of the patient) where the upper end of the stick is. This is not the point to be moxaed but serves merely as the midpoint (for further measuring). With a short, thin bamboo stick, measure as 1 *cun* the distance between the ends of the creases of the two middle finger joints. Use this (short) stick to measure 1 *cun* bilateral to the ink-marked point. These are the points.[2] Moxa them each with 5-7 cones but no more. Moxaing by this method never fails to effect a cure. These two points are where the heart vessel passes. All types of *yong* and *ju* disease are retention and stagnation of heart qi, thus giving rise to these kinds of toxins. Moxaing these frees the flow of the heart vessel and (consequently) results in safety and

---

[1] *Yong* refers to acute, localized, suppurative inflammatory lesions of the skin and subcutaneous tissues or the internal organs. *Ju* refers to suppurative inflammatory lesions of the subcutaneous tissues which are diffuse, flat swellings with overlying skin of normal color and absence of heat with little, if any, pain.

[2] These points are Diaphragm Shu (*Ge Shu*, Bl 17) and Liver Shu (*Gan Shu*, Bl 18).

instant healing. This may bring life back (even) to the dead. It is extraordinarily effective.

For sores growing all over the body: Pool at the Bend (*Qu Chi*, LI 11), Union Valley (*He Gu*, LI 4), (Leg) Three *Li* (*San Li*, St 36), Severed Bone (*Jue Gu*, GB 39), and Eye of the Knee (*Xi Yan*, St 35) [moxa 2 times 7 cones]

For swelling of the armpit and saber lumps[3]: Yang Assistance (*Yang Fu*, GB 38), Supreme Surge (*Tai Chong*, Liv 3), and Foot Overlooking Tears (*Zu Lin Qi*, GB 41)

For heat wind erratic papules: Shoulder Bone (*Jian Yu*, LI 15), Pool at the Bend (*Qu Chi*, LI 11), Marsh at the Bend (*Qu Ze*, Per 3), Jumping Round (*Huan Tiao*, GB 30), Union Valley (*He Gu*, LI 4), and Gushing Spring (*Yong Quan*, Ki 1)

For sore swelling with quivering with cold: Lesser Sea (*Shao Hai*, Ht 3)

For sores due to scabies and tinea: Pool at the Bend (*Qu Chi*, LI 11), Branch Ditch (*Zhi Gou*, TH 6), Yang Ravine (*Yang Xi*, LI 5), Yang Valley (*Yang Gu*, SI 5), Great Mound (*Da Ling*, Per 7), Union Valley (*He Gu*, LI 4), Back Ravine (*Hou Xi*, SI 3), Bend Middle (*Wei Zhong*, Bl 40), (Leg) Three *Li* (*San Li*, St 36), Yang Assistance (*Yang Fu*, GB 38), Kunlun (Mountain, *Kun Lun*, Bl 60), Moving Between (*Xing Jian*, Liv 2), Three Yin Intersection (*San Yin Jiao*, Sp 6), and Hundred Worm Burrow (*Bai Chong Wo, i.e.*, Sea of Blood [*Xue Hai*, Sp 10]), [*i.e.*, Eye of the Knee, *Xi Yan*, St 35]

---

3   Saber lumps refer to enlarged lymph nodes growing in or under the axillae.

For clove sores[4] growing on the face and around the corners of the mouth: Moxa Union Valley (*He Gu*, LI 4).

For clove sores growing on the hand: Pool at the Bend (*Qu Chi*, LI 11) [moxa]

For clove sores growing on the upper back: Shoulder Well (*Jian Jing*, GB 21), (Leg) Three *Li* (*San Li*, St 36), Bend Middle (*Wei Zhong*, Bl 40), (Foot) Overlooking Tears (*Lin Qi*, GB 41), Moving Between (*Xing Jian*, Liv 2), Connecting the Interior (*Tong Li*, Ht 5), Small Sea (*Xiao Hai*, SI 8), and Supreme Surge (*Tai Chong*, Liv 3)

For small and large scrofulous lumps: Lesser Sea (*Shao Hai*, Ht 3), [First insert the needle in the skin, and, after 36 respirations, push the needle into {the flesh}. Determine the depth of the insertion in accordance with the size of the lump's core, never letting it pass beyond {the size of} the core. Until after having turned {the needle} 33 {32 in a variant version; tr.} times, do not extract the needle.], Celestial Pool (*Tian Chi*, Per 1), Screen Gate (*Zhang Men*, Liv 13), (Foot) Overlooking Tears (*Lin Qi*, GB 41), Branch Ditch (*Zhi Gou*, TH 6), Yang Assistance (*Yang Fu*, GB 38) [moxa with 100 cones], Shoulder Well (*Jian Jing*, GB 21) [the same number of cones as years of age], and Arm Three *Li* (*Shou San Li*, LI 10)

Effusion (*i.e.*, breaking out) of *yong* and *ju* on the upper back: Shoulder Well (*Jian Jing*, GB 21) and Bend Middle (*Wei Zhong*, Bl 40). In addition, stick slices of garlic onto the sores and then moxa. If the sores are painless, moxa till they become painful. If they are painful, moxa them till they become painless. The more (cones are moxaed), the better.

---

4   Clove sores or toxins are a type of purulent sore which is hard and localized with a deep root.

The Category of Miscellaneous Diseases

F or the pulse in a person being faint and thin to such an extent that it disappears or appears sometimes but disappears at others: Puncture Recover Flow (*Fu Liu*, Ki 7) on the foot *shao yin* channel with a round-pointed, filiform needle to the depth of the bone. Direct the needle downward. Do not extract it till yang is recovered and the pulse is generated.

For scorpion sting and wounds caused by snake, dog, and centipede (bite) with unbearable pain: Needle against the flow of the affected channel(s) with (the patient) holding back their breath. Going counter to the flow of the channel(s) with the breath held back is to drain the toxic qi straight away. Breathing is undesirable because the toxic qi may otherwise penetrate the channel(s). The incantation (to be repeated) in the process of the needling is:

> Heaven is intelligent and the physician is honorable. They cherish the wish to safeguard longevity. The Supreme Mystery, which is unique, keeps to the true form, while the patron saints of the five viscera each safeguard the peace and calm of the viscera. Once the divine needle is inserted, all kinds of toxins must hide their forms hurriedly as under an imperial decree. This order is executed by the nine needles.

After reciting (this incantation) silently, blow one breath onto the needle, thinking that the needle should be likened to a firey dragon, and extract the disease from the heart and abdomen of the patient. Then healing will result soon.

119

For the drowned, who can be saved (only if it happened) overnight: Untie the belt of the dead person, and moxa Center of the Navel (*Qi Zhong, i.e.,* Spirit Gate, *Shen Que,* CV 8).

For rabid dog bite: Promptly moxa the wound at the bitten place.

For snake bite: Moxa the wound with 3 cones. Then stick a slice of garlic onto it and moxa over the garlic.

The Daily Locations of the Human God[1]

On the 1st day, (the human god) exists in the big toe in the *jue yin* phase. If it is needled, the instep will become swollen.

On the 2nd day, (the human god) exists in the lateral malleolus in the *shao yang* phase. If it is needled, the sinew channel will become slack.

On the 3rd day, (the human god) exists in the medial aspect of the thigh in the *shao yin* phase. If it is needled, there arises lower abdominal pain.

On the 4th day, (the human god) exists in the lumbus in the *tai yang* phase. If it is needled, the lumbus will become stooped and weak.

On the 5th day, (the human god) exists in the mouth in the *tai yin* phase. If it is needled or moxaed, the tongue will become stiff.

---

[1] *Ren shen* or human god refers to one of several personal spirits believed by traditional Asian doctors to inhabit and to move around the body based on certain cycles of time. In this case, this personal spirit inhabits a different body part each day of the lunar month. Therefore, for fear of injuring this personal spirit, needling and, in some cases, moxibustion is forbidden at those places on those days. Of the various methods of divining the locations of these personal spirits, the locations for the days of the lunar month are the easiest to remember and use and the most important in traditional practice.

On the 6th day, (the human god) exists in the hands in the *yang ming* phase. If it is needled, the throat will become inhibited.

On the 7th day, (the human god) exists in the inner malleolus in the *shao yin* phase. If it is needled or moxaed, the sinews of the yin channels will become tense.

On the 8th day, (the human god) exists in the wrists in the *tai yang* phase. If it is needled or moxaed, the wrist will become unable to contract.

On the 9th day, (the human god) exists in the coccyx in the *jue yin* phase. If it is needled or moxaed, the disease will become urgent (*i.e.*, acute).

On the 10th day, (the human god) exists in the upper and lower back in the *tai yin* phase. If it is needled or moxaed, the upper and lower back will become stooped.

On the 11th day, (the human god) exists in the nose pillar in the *yang ming* phase. If it is needled or moxaed, the teeth and face will become swollen.

On the 12th day, (the human god) exists in the hairline in the *shao yang* phase. If it is needled or moxaed, the person will be caused impaired hearing.

On the 13th day, (the human god) exists in the teeth in the *shao yin* phase. If it is needled or moxaed, qi will become cold.

On the 14th day, (the human god) exists in the venter in the *yang ming* phase. If it is needled, there will arise qi swelling.

On the 15th day, (the human god) exists throughout the body and it is inappropriate either to supplement or drain. Either needling or moxaing is absolutely prohibited.

On the 16th day, (the human god) exists in the chest in the *tai yin* phase. If it is needled, there will arise counterflow breathing (*i.e.*, dyspnea).

On the 17th day, (the human god) exists in the qi thoroughfare (*i.e.*, groin) in the *yang ming* phase. If it is needled, there will arise difficulty breathing.

On the 18th day, (the human god) exists in the medial aspects of the thighs in the *shao yin* phase. If it is needled, there will arise qi pain giving a dragging discomfort to the genitals.

On the 19th day, (the human god) exists in the insteps in the *yang ming* phase. If it is moxaed (the undesired effect is left out from the original text; tr.).

On the 20th day, (the human god) exists in the inner malleolus in the *shao yin* phase. If it is needled, there will arise hypertonicity of the channel sinews.

On the 21st day, (the human god) exists in the small fingers of the hands in the *tai yang* phase. If it is needled, the hands will become insensitive.

On the 22nd day, (the human god) exists in the lateral malleolus in the *shao yang* phase. If it is needled, the channel sinews will become slack.

On the 23rd day, (the human god) exists in the lumbus and feet in the *jue yin* phase. If it is needled, spasms will be occasioned.

On the 24th day, (the human god) exists in the hands in the *yang ming* phase. If it is needled, the throat will become inhibited.

On the 25th day, (the human god) exists in the feet in the *yang ming* phase. If it is needled, there will arise distention of stomach qi.

On the 26th day, (the human god) exists in the chest in the *tai yin* phase. If it is needled or moxaed, there will arise dyspnea and coughing.

On the 27th day, (the human god) exists in the knees in the *yang ming* phase. If it is needled, there will arise counterflow inversion along the foot channels.

On the 28th day, (the human god) exists in the genitals in the *shao yin* phase. If it is needled, there will arise acute lower abdominal pain.

On the 29th day, (the human god) exists in the knees in the *jue yin* phase. If it is needled, the sinews will become atonic and weak.

On the 30th day, (the human god) exists in the insteps in the *yang ming* phase. If it is needled, the stomach qi will be damaged.

In reference to the department of acupuncture and moxibustion, although there are the *(Zhen Jiu) Zi Shen Jing (Life-fostering Classic of Acupuncture & Moxibustion)*[2], the *Zhen Jiu Si Shu (The Four Books of Acupuncture & Moxibustion)*[3] (and others), their contents

---

[2]   The *Zhen Jiu Zi Shen Jing* is a work by Wang Zhi-zhong of the Song dynasty which was first published in 1220 CE.

[3]   The *Zhen Jiu Si Shu*, which was compiled by Dou Gui-fang in 1311 CE, includes the *Huang Di Ming Tang Jiu Jing (The Yellow Emperor's Ming Tang Moxibustion Classic)* by an anonymous author, the *Jiu Gao Huang Shu Fa (The Gao Huang Moxa Method Book)* by Zhuang Zhuo of the Song dynasty,

are too vast and voluminous (for readers) to peer into their wonderful essentials. Elder-born Chen Hong-gang, whose work is the only exception, came into possession of the secrets handed down in the family of the Reverend (Xi) Zi-sang and collected all the essentials into a book for later students to learn. Now it has undergone collation and has been made (more) compact, more pertinent, and pithy. Thus all later generations under heaven will be helped into a realm of humanity and longevity.

The End of the *Shen Ying Jing*

Propitious Day, the 5th month, the second year of the reign of Seiho[4]
Tsuruyacho, Nijo[5], (Japan)
printed by Tahara Jinsaemon

---

the *Zi Wu Liu Zhu Zhen Jing (Acupuncture Classic of Midday/Midnight Point Selection)* by He Ruo-yu of the Jin dynasty, and the *Zhen Jiu Zhi Nan (A Guide to Acupuncture & Moxibustion)* by Dou Jie of the Yuan dynasty.

4   Seiho was a Japanese emperor who ruled over the country from 1644-47 CE.

5   A place in Kyoto, Japan

Added Treatment Methods

Treatise on Wind Stroke
From Master Xu's Book[1]

In terms of wind stroke, there are five signs indicating incurability. Open mouth, shut eyes, fecal incontinence, enuresis, and thunderous rale in the throat are all malign signs. Furthermore, wind stroke is the chief of the hundreds of diseases, and its changes and transformations are various. (Wind) may strike either the viscera or the bowels. Phlegm or qi, anger or joy may give it the advantage of a loophole to play havoc. If it strikes the viscera, it causes people to lose consciousness of human affairs with phlegm and drool congestion and blocking, thunderous rale in the throat, paralysis of the limbs, insensitivity to pain, and sluggish or difficult speech. Therefore, it is difficult to treat. If it strikes the bowels, it causes people hemiplegia with deviated eyes and mouth, sensibility to pain and itching, ability to speak, and normal complexion and form. Thus, it is easy to treat.

To treat wind stroke, one should first study its patterns before performing needling. The patterns each have their particular names in terms of their manifestations when the five viscera and six bowels are struck. It is necessary first to find out the origin and name of the pattern and then perform needling in accor-

---

[1] This refers to the *Zhen Jiu Da Quan* (*Comprehensive Collection of Acupuncture & Moxibustion*) by Xu Feng of the Ming dynasty.

127

dance with (the condition of) the root and branch. This never fails to bring effect.

1. Liver stroke displays (the manifestations of) absence of sweating and aversion to cold. Its color (*i.e.*, the color of the patient's complexion) is green-blue. It is (also) called anger stroke.

2. Heart stroke displays (the manifestations of) copious sweating and susceptibility to fright. Its color is red. It is (also) called thought-worry stroke.

3. Spleen stroke displays (the manifestations of) copious sweating and body heat. Its color is yellow. It is (also) called joy stroke.

4. Lung stroke displays (the manifestations of) copious sweating and aversion to wind. Its color is white. It is (also) called qi stroke.

5. Kidney stroke displays (the manifestations of) copious sweating and body cold. Its color is black. It is (also) called qi taxation stroke.

6. Stomach stroke displays (the manifestations of) inability to take in drink and food and phlegm and drool congestion in the upper. Its color is light yellow. It is (also) called after-meal stroke.

7. Gallbladder stroke displays (the manifestations of) heavy eyes and fast (*i.e.*, long) sleeping without waking. Its color is green. It is (also) called fright stroke.

Needling Methods for the Emergency Treatment of the Initial Stage of Wind Stroke From the *Qian Kun Sheng Yi*[1]

A t the initial stage of wind stroke with collapse, sudden cloudedness, congesting and stagnated phlegm and drool, loss of consciousness of human affairs, tightly clenched jaw, and inability to take medicinal decoctions, promptly prick with a three-edged needle the twelve well points on the fingers. It is necessary to remove the malign blood. Moreover, to treat all malign patterns of sudden death, unconsciousness of human affairs, and intestine-gripping *sha*[2], this is a miraculous technique to bring back life to the dead. Lesser Shang (*Shao Shang*, Lu 11), two points; Shang Yang (*Shang Yang*, LI 1), two points; Central Hub (*Zhong Chong*, Per 9), two points; Passage Hub (*Guan Chong*, TH 1), two points; Lesser Surge (*Shao Chong*, Ht 9), two points; and Lesser Marsh (*Shao Ze*, SI 1), two points.

---

[1] The *Qian Kun Sheng Yi (For the Purpose of Life[-Securing Between] Qian [i.e., Heaven] & Kun [i.e., Earth])* was compiled by Zhu Quan in 1391 CE. It is a very concise yet all-encompassing book, touching on nearly all the fields of TCM and acumoxatherapy.

[2] Intestine-gripping *sha*, also known as dry sudden turmoil, is a pattern which manifests with gripping abdominal pain, dry retching, desire yet inability to evacuate stools, vexation and agitation, and, in extreme cases, a green-blue facial complexion, massive sweating, and an absence of the pulse.

The Secret Technique of Acupuncture & Moxibustion for Wind Stroke Paralysis From the *Qian Kun Sheng Yi*

F or wind stroke (with) deviated eyes and mouth: Auditory Convergence (*Ting Hui*, GB 2), Jawbone (*Jia Che*, St 6), and Earth Granary (*Di Cang*, St 4)

In the case of deviation to the left, it is appropriate to moxa the right (side). In the case of deviation to the right, it is appropriate to moxa the left (side). Moxa the depressions in the center of the deviations, each with 2 times 7 cones the size of grains of wheat. Moxa in quick succession till all the wind qi is removed and the eyes and mouth are back in (their proper) position.

A (special) method: Insert a 5 *cun* long writing-brush holder in the ear, caulking flour dough around the holder. Moxa at the outer end of the bamboo tube (*i.e.*, the brush holder) with 2 times 7 cones. Moxa the left for deviation on the right, and moxa the right for deviation on the left.

For wind stroke with wind evils having entered the bowels causing paralysis of the hand and foot: Hundred Convergences (*Bai Hui*, GV 20), the hairline anterior to the ear, Shoulder Bone (*Jian Yu*, LI 15), Pool at the Bend (*Qu Chi*, LI 11), Wind Market (*Feng Shi*, GB 31), Leg Three *Li* (*Zu San Li*, St 36), and Severed Bone (*Jue Gu*, GB 39). Whenever the extremities feel numb and insensitive or have an enduring pain, these being the signs of wind evils having entered the bowels, it is appropriate to moxa the (above) seven points. Moxa the right for disease on the left, and moxa the left for disease on the right until the wind qi is reduced and relieved.

For wind stroke with wind evils having entered the viscera giving rise to qi block and drool congestion, loss of speech, and critical cloudedness: Hundred Convergences (*Bai Hui*, GV 20), Great Vertebra (*Da Zhui*, GV 14), Wind Pool (*Feng Chi*, GB 20), Shoulder Well (*Jian Jing*, GB 21), Pool at the Bend (*Qu Chi*, LI 11), Leg Three *Li* (*Zu San Li*, St 36), and Intermediary Courier (*Jian Shi*, Per 5). Whenever the sensation of vexation and agitation in the heart arises with gloomy spirit and thought or stubborn numbness of the extremities, these being signs of wind evils having entered the viscera, moxa without delay the above seven points each with 5 times 7 cones. (Although) the wind (may) not (seem) threatening, in the two seasons of spring and autumn, it is necessary to moxa these seven points to drain wind qi. One should particularly take care of people who have been possessed of wind.

For wind stroke (with) nasal congestion and loss of smell, frequent running of clear nasal mucus, and ambilateral or hemilateral head wind, for white scales growing (on the skin), and for fright epilepsy with upturned eyes and inability to recognize people: Fontanel Meeting (*Xin Hui*, GV 22) [moxa]

For wind stroke (with) swelling of the skin on the head, visual dizziness and double vision, shivering with (alternating) cold and heat, and sore eyes without ability to see far: Upper Star (*Shang Xing*, GV 23) [needle {or} moxa]

For wind stroke, wind epilepsy, tugging and slackening, etc.: Hall of Impression (*Yin Tang*, M-HN-3) [needle {or} moxa]

For wind stroke (with) hypertonicity of the head and nape of the neck and inability to look round: Wind Mansion (*Feng Fu*, GV 16) [needle]

For wind stroke with inability to lift the hands: Yang Pool (*Yang Chi*, TH 4) [needle {or} moxa]

For wind stroke with aching of and inability to bend or stretch the wrist and pain in and inability to hold things with the fingers: Outer Pass (*Wai Guan*, TH 5) [needle {or} moxa]

For wind stroke with weakness, insensitivity, and contracture of the hand: Arm Three *Li* (*Shou San Li*, LI 10) [needle {or} moxa]

For wind stroke with phlegmatic coughing, hypertonicity of the elbow, cold and heat, and fright epilepsy: Broken Sequence (*Lie Que*, Lu 7) [needle {or} moxa]

For wind stroke with susceptibility to fright and fearfulness, loss of voice, and aching pain in the elbow and wrist: Connecting the Interior (*Tong Li*, Ht 5) [needle {or} moxa]

For wind stroke with aching pain in the lumbus and crotch, inability to turn (the body) over, and dragging (discomfort) between the lumbus and the lateral costal region: Jumping Round (*Huan Tiao*, GB 30) [needle {or} moxa]

For wind stroke with cramps and hypertonicity (of the leg with) weakness and pain in walking: Kunlun (Mountain, *Kun Lun*, Bl 60) [needle {or} moxa]

For wind stroke with numbness and insensitivity of the foot and leg with cold *bi* and cold pain: Yang Mound (Spring) (*Yang Ling*, GB 34) [needle {or} moxa]

For wind stroke with hypertonicity of the upper and lower back: Bend Middle (*Wei Zhong*, Bl 40) [needle]

For wind stroke with aching pain in the foot and knee with cramps and hypertonicity (of the leg): Mountain Support (*Cheng Shan*, Bl 57) [needle {or} moxa]

To treat vacuity detriment and the five taxations and seven damages[1], the key points are Kiln Path (*Tao Dao*, GV 13), 1 point, moxa with 2 times 7 cones; Body Pillar (*Shen Zhu*, GV 12), 1 point, moxa with 2 times 7 cones; Lung *Shu* (*Fei Shu*, Bl 13), 2 points, moxa with 7 times 7 or up to 100 cones; Gao Huang (*Gao Huang*, Bl 43), 2 points, moxa with 3 times 7 or up to 7 times 7 cones.

---

[1] Vacuity detriment can be a collective term for the five taxations and seven damages. In a strict sense, however, it refers to the four types of vacuity, *i.e.*, qi, blood, yin, and yang vacuities, which are caused by the seven affects, taxation fatigue, dietary irregularity, injury by alcohol and sex, and neglect of one's health.

The five taxations are heart, lung, spleen, kidney, and liver taxations. The five taxations may also refer to injuries due to prolonged viewing, prolonged sitting, prolonged lying, prolonged standing, and prolonged walking.

The seven damages are overeating damaging the spleen; great anger damaging the liver; weight-lifting and long staying on damp ground damaging the kidneys; cold evil and water rheum damaging the lungs; worry, thought, and anxiety damaging the heart; wind, rain, summerheat, and winter cold damaging the form; and fright and terror damaging the will.

Cold Damage
From the *Ju Ying*[1]

F ever is due to wind cold lodging in the skin and the yang qi being confined and oppressed. This is exterior heat. When the yang qi sinks into the yin phase to steam and fume, this is interior heat.

For sweat refusing to exude and aversion to cold as after a soaking: Jade Pillow (*Yu Zhen*, Bl 9), Great Shuttle (*Da Zhu*, Bl 11), Liver *Shu* (*Gan Shu*, Bl 18), Diaphragm *Shu* (*Ge Shu*, Bl 17), and Kiln Path (*Tao Dao*, GV 13)

For body heat and aversion to cold: Back Ravine (*Hou Xi*, SI 3)

For body heat, sweating, and inversion frigidity of the feet: Great Metropolis (*Da Du*, Sp 2)

For body heat, headache, and inability to take in food: Triple Heater *Shu* (*San Jiao Shu*, Bl 22)

For sweat refusing to exude: Union Valley (*He Gu*, LI 4), Back Ravine (*Hou Xi*, SI 3), Yang Pool (*Yang Chi*, TH 4), Severe Mouth (*Li Dui*, St 45), Ravine Divide (*Jie Xi*, St 41), and Wind Pool (*Feng Chi*, GB 20)

For body heat with dyspnea: Third Space (*San Jian*, LI 3)

---

[1] The full name of this book is the *Zhen Jiu Ju Ying (Gatherings from Acupuncture & Moxibustion Works)*. It is an important work in this art compiled by Gao Wu and published in 1529 CE.

For persistent remaining heat: Pool at the Bend (*Qu Chi*, LI 11)

For vexation, fullness, and sweat refusing to exude: Wind Pool (*Feng Chi*, GB 20) and Life Gate (*Ming Men*, GV 4)

For cold and heat (despite) sweat exuding: Fifth Place (*Wu Chu*, Bl 5), Bamboo Gathering (*Zan Zhu*, Bl 2), and Upper Venter (*Shang Wan*, CV 13)

For vexation of the heart and frequent retching: Great Tower Gate (*Ju Que*, CV 14) and Shang Hill (*Shang Qiu*, Sp 5)

For body heat, headache, and sweat refusing to exude: Spring at the Bend (*Qu Quan*, Liv 8)

For advancing and retreating (*i.e.*, intermittent) body heat and headache: Spirit Pass (*Shen Dao*, GV 11), Origin Pass (*Guan Yuan*, CV 4), and Suspended Skull (*Xuan Lu*, GB 5)

The above can be found in the *Zhen Jing* (*Classic of Needling*, a.k.a. the *Ling Shu* or *Spiritual Pivot*)

For all the six pulses being deep and thin, coming on (*i.e.*, beating) 2-3 times for one respiration: Sea of Qi (*Qi Hai*, CV 6) [moxa] and Origin Pass (*Guan Yuan*, CV 4) [moxa]

For *shao yin* fever[2]: Great Ravine (*Tai Xi*, Ki 3) [moxa]. Aversion to cold is started from yang in the case of existence of heat but from yin in the case of absence of heat.

---

2   In cold damage, the *shao yin* pattern can be of two types, the nonheat pattern and the heat pattern. The latter is characterized by vexation, insomnia, dry throat, red tongue tip, diarrhea, and coughing.

For the upper back averse to cold with an (agreeable) taste in the mouth: Origin Pass (*Guan Yuan*, CV 4)

Aversion to wind presents itself as wind stroke damaging the defensive in the presence of sweating, but as cold damaging the constructive in the absence of sweating. (For these,) first needle Wind Mansion (*Feng Fu*, GV 16) and Wind Pool (*Feng Chi*, GB 20) and then drink *Gui Zhi Ge Gen Tang* (Cinnamon & Pueraria Decoction).[3]

In the case of chest and flank fullness with delirious speech, evil qi first damages the exterior and then the interior and further enters the heart. (For it:) Cycle Gate (*Qi Men*, Liv 14)

Chest bind is blocking of the visceral qi which is stopped from flowing and spreading. That which gives pain when pressed is a minor bind and that which is painful (all the time even) when not pressed is a major bind. (For these:) Cycle Gate (*Qi Men*, Liv 14) [needle] and Lung *Shu* (*Fei Shu*, Bl 13) [needle]

For chest bind due to blood with heat penetrating the blood chamber[4] in women: Cycle Gate (*Qi Men*, Liv 14) [needle]. In addition, make a cake of Rhizoma Coptidis Chinensis (*Huang Lian*) and 7 pieces of Semen Crotonis Tiglii (*Ba Dou*), put it over the navel, and moxa on it until a bowel movement is induced.

---

[3]   This decoction is composed of Radix Puerariae Lobatae (*Ge Gen*), Radix Albus Paeoniae Lactiflorae (*Bai Shao*), Ramulus Cinnamomi (*Gui Zhi*), fresh Rhizoma Zingiberis (*Sheng Jiang*), and Radix Glycyrrhizae (*Gan Cao*).

[4]   The blood chamber may refer to either the penetrating vessel or the uterus.

For counterflow coughing due to disconnection of qi in the chest with a noise as a result of the contention between water and fire: Cycle Gate (*Qi Men*, Liv 14)

Lower abdominal fullness may be due to qi in the upper (or) urine in the lower. Because they fail to be discharged when they ought, they accumulate to give rise to fullness or acute pain in the abdomen. (For this,) needle Bend Middle (*Wei Zhong*, Bl 40) or the Snatching-Life-Back point and other places.[5]

Vexation and agitation are due to evil qi in the interior. Vexation is unrest occurring in the internal, and agitation is unrest occurring in the external. Six to seven days after (contraction of) cold damage, if the pulse is faint with inversion frigidity of the extremities and there is vexation and agitation, moxa *Jue Yin Shu* (*Jue Yin Shu*, Bl 14).

Blood amassment is static blood caused by heat toxins flowing downward. The *shao yin* pattern (with) diarrhea with blood and pus in the stools allows for needling. The *yang ming* pattern manifests with blood in the stools and delirious speech. (In this case,) heat has invariably entered the blood chamber with sweat exuding (merely) on the head. (The point to) needle is Cycle Gate (*Qi Men*, Liv 14).

Retching and vomiting is due to exterior evils transmitting into the interior. When the interior qi counterflows upward, there arises retching and vomiting. In the case of an (agreeable) taste in the mouth with a faint, choppy, and weak pulse, moxa *Jue Yin* (*Jue Yin*, Bl 14).

---

5   This point may be *Gao Huang Shu* (*Gao Huang Shu*, Bl 43), and the other places implied may refer to Sea of Qi (*Qi Hai*, CV 6), Origin Pass (*Guan Yuan*, CV 4), Stone Gate (*Shi Men*, CV 5), Central Pole (*Zhong Ji*, CV 3), and (Leg) Three *Li* (*San Li*, St 36).

As to throbbing and shivering, throbbing indicates that the righteous qi is becoming triumphant, while shivering indicates that evil qi is becoming triumphant. When evil contends with the righteous, heart throbbing with shivering externally shows the disease to be on the point of resolution. If the evil qi is superabundant internally and the righteous qi is overly vacuous, the heart shivers with jaws chattering. If the body does not tremble, cold counterflow will result later. (For it,) moxa Fish Border (*Yu Ji*, Lu 10).

Counterflow of the four is counterflow frigidity of the limbs. Coolness may accumulate to develop into cold, and the qi of the six bowels is made to expire externally. Counterflow cold of the feet and lower legs (is ascribed to) the *shao yin*, while body cold to the *jue yin*. (For these,) moxa Sea of Qi (*Qi Hai*, CV 6), Kidney *Shu* (*Shen Shu*, Bl 23), and Liver *Shu* (*Gan Shu*, Bl 18).

Inversion is counterflow frigidity of the extremities with yang qi depressed and sunken. Because heat qi counterflows and is depressed, the hands and feet become frigid. (For this,) needle Inner Court (*Nei Ting*, St 44) and Great Metropolis (*Da Du*, Sp 2). If the pulse is skipping in inversion, moxa these.

As to oppression and cloudedness, oppression is obstruction of qi, while cloudedness is unclear spirit, *i.e.*, stupor. In most cases, it is a result of extreme vacuity taken advantage of by cold or is caused by vomiting and diarrhea. To treat the *tai yang* and *shao yang* combination disease[6] of headache or cloudedness and oppression as in chest bind, needle Great Vertebra (*Da Zhui*, GV

---

6   This combination disease is comprised of both the *tai yang* pattern of headache and fever and the *shao yang* pattern of bitter taste in the mouth, dry throat, and visual dizziness. In extreme cases, there may be vomiting above and diarrhea below, abdominal urgency with rectal pressure, and burning heat in the anus.

14), Lung *Shu* (*Fei Shu*, Bl 13), and Liver *Shu* (*Gan Shu*, Bl 18). Do not promote sweating in any event.

Self-diarrhea is duck-stool diarrhea or loose bowels not due to offensive precipitation. If the pulse is slightly choppy with retching and sweating, (one) is bound to change clothes.[7] If, contrarily, one does not (change clothes) frequently, it is necessary to warm the upper by moxaing in order to eliminate yin. If the urination is uninhibited with heat rather than cold in the hands and the pulse not coming on, moxa Great Ravine (*Tai Xi*, Ki 3).

The *shao yin* (pattern) with loose bowels with blood in the stool necessitates needling. It is proper to use the common (point, *i.e.*, Great Ravine, *Tai Xi*, Ki 3).

Sudden turmoil is vomiting above and diarrhea below with extravagant perturbation and glaring tumult. The evil is in the middle heater with the stomach qi being out of order and yin and yang at odds and separated. Therefore, there arises vomiting above and diarrhea below with agitation, unrest, vexation, and disturbance. (This may also give rise to) dry sudden turmoil or a gripping or stabbing abdominal pain (instead. For all of these,) needle Bend Middle (*Wei Zhong*, Bl 40) and the Snatching-Life-Back point.

In relation to abdominal pain, there may be repletion or vacuity, cold or heat, (possibly) with dry stools and old accumulation. Lack of pain under pressure indicates vacuity, while pressure (exacerbating) the pain indicates repletion. Both need moxibustion. If not moxaed, the patient will be left to have cold bind which, over time, will make more trouble. If qi upsurges into the

---

[7] Changing clothes means going to the latrine and thus implies diarrhea.

heart, death will be caused. (For this,) needle Bend Middle (*Wei Zhong*, Bl 40).

The yin pattern of yin toxins is a disease of yin exuberance with faint yang wasted above. Therefore, there arises heaviness (of the body), counterflow frigidity of the limbs, pounding periumbilical pain, and counterflow inversion or frigidity with the six pulses deep and thin. (For this,) moxa Origin Pass (*Guan Yuan*, CV 4) and Sea of Qi (*Qi Hai*, CV 6).

For *tai yang* and *shao yang* combination disease: Needle Lung *Shu* (*Fei Shu*, Bl 13) and Liver *Shu* (*Gan Shu*, Bl 18). In case of headache, needle Great Vertebra (*Da Zhui*, GV 14).

Inhibited voiding of urine is due to evil accumulating in the internal and keeping fluids and humor from flowing. In case of block below with severe yin cold, moxa.

For the yin pattern of inhibited urination with the testicles withdrawn into the lower abdomen and deadly pain: Moxa Stone Gate (*Shi Men*, CV 5).

Insensitivity is lack of moderateness and harmony (with no sense of) itching, pain, cold, or heat. When the righteous qi is blocked and subjugated by evil qi, depressed and unable to dissipate, blood and qi become vacuous and short. This results in (insensitivity). Take, (for instance, Qin) Yue-ren.[8] He examined the Prince of Guo[9] and determined his deathlike inversion was curable based on (his) depression, cloudedness, and insensitivity.

---

[8]   This is Qin Yue-ren, more commonly known as Bian Que (*circa* 5th-4th century BCE) who has been acclaimed as the forefather of pulse examination and formulary in TCM for scores of centuries.

[9]   Guo was a small state in the Warring States period (475-221 BCE).

(Because of this, his) needling effected a cure. (Such a) diagnosis is made (only) by a divine physician. If the pulse had been floating and surging with sweat like oil with incessant gasping and generalized insensitivity, how could (Qin) Yue-ren have been able to treat it?

All the above can be found in the *Shang Han Zhi Li (Illustrations of the Treatment of Cold Damage)* by Master Liu.[10]

---

[10] Master Liu was Liu Chun, who lived between the Yuan and Ming dynasties and whose father was a disciple of the preeminent TCM physician and scholar Zhu Zhen-heng (a.k.a. Dan-xi). Besides the *Shang Han Zhi Li*, he left many other works, including the *Yi Jing Xiao Xue (An Etymological Study of the Medical Classics)* and the *Za Bing Zhi Li (Illustrations of the Treatment of Miscellaneous Diseases)*. Yang Ji-zhou in his *Zhen Jiu Da Cheng* drew a lot upon these two sources.

Miscellaneous Diseases

Wind largely governs blood vacuity, qi vacuity, fire, and dampness as well as copious phlegm.

For wind stroke: Spirit Gate (*Shen Que*, CV 8), Wind Pool (*Feng Chi*, GB 20), Hundred Convergences (*Bai Hui*, GV 20), Pool at the Bend (*Qu Chi*, LI 11), Wind Screen (*Yi Feng*, TH 17), Wind Market (*Feng Shi*, GB 31), Jumping Round (*Huan Tiao*, GB 30), and Shoulder Bone (*Jian Yu*, LI 15). All of the above can be moxaed to course wind (or) needled to conduct qi.

For cold, refer to Cold Damage.

For cold genitals with (yang qi) sunken and expiring pulses, it is appropriate to moxa.

Fever is classified into tidal heat with cold, distressed heat, and intermittent heat.

For heat disease with sweat refusing to exude: Shang Yang (*Shang Yang*, LI 1), Union Valley (*He Gu*, LI 4), Yang Valley (*Yang Gu*, SI 5), Pinched Ravine (*Xia Xi*, GB 43), Severe Mouth (*Li Dui*, St 45), Palace of Toil (*Lao Gong*, Per 8), and Wrist Bone (*Wan Gu*, SI 4). (These) serve the end of conducting qi.

For heat beyond measure and incessant sweating: Sunken Valley (*Xian Gu*, St 43). (This) serves the end of draining heat.

Abdominal pain may be due to vacuity, repletion, cold, qi stagnation, dead blood, accumulated heat, wind dampness, phlegm fright, phlegm food, sores, *sha*, and *shan*.

Repletion (abdominal) pain requires draining (at) Supreme Surge (*Tai Chong*, Liv 3), Supreme White (*Tai Bai*, Sp 3), Great Abyss (*Tai Yuan*, Lu 9), Great Mound (*Da Ling*, Per 7), and Three Yin Intersection (*San Yin Jiao*, Sp 6).

If evils lodge in the channels and connecting vessels and medicinals are not able to reach them, it is appropriate to moxa Sea of Qi (*Qi Hai*, CV 6), Origin Pass (*Guan Yuan*, CV 4), and Central Venter (*Zhong Wan*, CV 12).

Headache may be due to wind, wind heat, phlegm, dampness, and cold. True headache with green-blue (*i.e.*, cyanotic) complexion of the hands and feet reaching to the wrists and ankles ends in death without a remedy. Moxibustion can course and dissipate cold. As for acupuncture, in the case of a floating pulse, needle Wrist Bone (*Wan Gu*, SI 4) and Capital Bone (*Jing Gu*, Bl 64). In the case of a long pulse, needle Union Valley (*He Gu*, LI 4) and Surging Yang (*Chong Yang*, St 42). In the case of a bowstring pulse, needle Yang Pool (*Yang Chi*, TH 4), Wind Mansion (*Feng Fu*, GV 16), and Wind Pool (*Feng Chi*, GB 20).

Lumbago may be due to qi vacuity, blood vacuity, kidney disease, wind dampness, damp heat, (blood) stasis, cold, and qi stagnation.

In the case of blood stagnated below, needle Bend Middle (*Wei Zhong*, Bl 40) [let out blood] and moxa Kidney *Shu* (*Shen Shu*, Bl 23) and Kunlun (Mountain, *Kun Lun*, Bl 60). In addition, obtain Apex Radicis Praeparati Aconiti Carmichaeli (*Fu Zi Jian*), Apex Radicis Aconiti (*Wu Tou Jian*), Rhizoma Arisaematis (*Nan Xing*), Secretio Moschi Moschiferi (*She Xiang*), Realgar (*Xiong Huang*), Camphora (*Zhang Nao*), and Flos Caryophylii (*Ding Xiang*) and make these into pills with heated honey. Dissolve them in Succus Zingiberis (*Jiang Zhi*, to form) a paste and rub (the painful place) with it in the palm after heating it.

Lateral costal pain (may be due to) exuberant liver fire and wood qi repletion which (in turn) may be caused by dead blood, stasis pouring, and tense liver. (For it,) needle Hill Homeland (*Qiu Xu*, GB 40) and Central River (*Zhong Du*, GB 32).

Heart pain may be due to wind cold, qi and blood vacuity, and accumulated food heat. (For it,) needle Great Ravine (*Tai Xi*, Ki 3), Blazing Valley (*Ran Gu*, Ki 2), Cubit Marsh (*Chi Ze*, Lu 5), Moving Between (*Xing Jian*, Liv 2), Interior Strengthening (*Jian Li*, CV 11), Great Metropolis (*Da Du*, Sp 2), Supreme White (*Tai Bai*, Sp 3), Central Venter (*Zhong Wan*, CV 12), Spirit Gate (*Shen Men*, Ht 7), and Gushing Spring (*Yong Quan*, Ki 1).

Toothache is governed by blood heat, heat existing in the stomach opening, wind cold, damp heat, and worm eating (*i.e.*, tooth decay. For it,) needle Union Valley (*He Gu*, LI 4), Inner Court (*Nei Ting*, St 44), Floating White (*Fu Bai*, GB 10), Yang White (*Yang Bai*, GB 14), and Third Space (*San Jian*, LI 3).

Eye (disorders) are governed by liver qi repletion, wind heat, phlegm heat, blood stasis heat, blood repletion, and qi congestion. (For them,) needle Upper Star (*Shang Xing*, GV 23), Hundred Convergences (*Bai Hui*, GV 20), Spirit Court (*Shen Ting*, GV 24), Before the Vertex (*Qian Ding*, GV 21), Bamboo Gathering (*Zan Zhu*, Bl 2), and Silk Bamboo Hole (*Si Zhu Kong*, TH 23). (They) diffuse and drain (heat and repletion). For pain (in the eyes,) needle Wind Pool (*Feng Chi*, GB 20) and Union Valley (*He Gu*, LI 4). (The points that) Zhang Zi-he[1] chose to treat the eyes are Spirit Court (*Shen Ting*, GV 24), Upper Star (*Shang Xing*, GV 23), and Before the Vertex (*Qian Ding*, GV 21).

---

[1] Zhang Zi-he, a.k.a Zhang Cong-zheng (*circa* 1156-1228 CE), was one of the four great masters of the Jin/Yuan dynasties. He was the founder of the *Gong Xia Pai* (School of Attack & Precipitation).

For great cold offending the brain and affecting and sending pain to the eyes or contention between wind and dampness giving rise to (eye) screen: Moxa Second Space (*Er Jian*, LI 2) and Union Valley (*He Gu*, LI 4).

For *gan* eyes[2] in children: Moxa Union Valley (*He Gu*, LI 4) [2 points] each with 1 cone.

Diarrhea and dysentery (may be due to) qi vacuity with cold and heat, food accumulation, wind evil, fright evil, heat dampness, sunken yang qi, and phlegm accumulation. They should be treated in accordance (with specific patterns. Comparatively speaking,) diarrhea is moderate, while dysentery is severe.

For sunken (yang qi): Moxa Spleen *Shu* (*Pi Shu*, Bl 20), Origin Pass (*Guan Yuan*, CV 4), Kidney *Shu* (*Shen Shu*, Bl 23), Recover Flow (*Fu Liu*, Ki 7), Abdominal Lament (*Fu Ai*, Sp 16), Long Strong (*Chang Qiang*, GV 1), Great Ravine (*Tai Xi*, Ki 3), (Leg) Three *Li* (*San Li*, St 36), Qi Abode (*Qi She*, St 11), Central Venter (*Zhong Wan*, CV 12), and Large Intestine *Shu* (*Da Chang Shu*, Bl 25).

For white dysentery: Moxa Large Intestine *Shu* (*Da Chang Shu*, Bl 25).

For red dysentery: Moxa Small Intestine *Shu* (*Xiao Chang Shu*, Bl 27).

---

[2] *Gan* is primarily a pediatric condition. Its main symptom is increasing emaciation in spite of large food intake. Its other clinical manifestations include a yellow facial complexion, thinning, brittle hair, enlarged belly with prominent green-blue veins, and lethargy. If it develops to affect the eyes, it is called *gan* eyes.

Malaria is classified into wind summerheat, mountain forest miasma, old food malaria[3], malaria mother[4], cold damp *bi*, malaria of the five viscera, and malaria of the five bowels. (For all these,) needle Union Valley (*He Gu*, LI 4), Pool at the Bend (*Qu Chi*, LI 11), and Offspring of the Noble (*Gong Sun*, Sp 4). First needle and then moxa the vertebra immediately under Great Hammer (*Da Zhui*, GV 14) with 3 times 7 cones.

Coughing may be due to wind, cold, fire, taxation, phlegm, lung distention, and dampness. (For it,) moxa Celestial Chimney (*Tian Tu*, CV 22), Lung *Shu* (*Fei Shu*, Bl 13), Shoulder Well (*Jian Jing*, GB 21), Lesser Shang (*Shao Shang*, Lu 11), Blazing Valley (*Ran Gu*, Ki 2), Liver *Shu* (*Gan Shu*, Bl 18), Cycle Gate (*Qi Men*, Liv 14), Moving Between (*Xing Jian*, Liv 2), Ridge Spring (*Lian Quan*, CV 23), and Protuberance Assistant (*Fu Tu*, LI 18), and needle Marsh at the Bend (*Qu Ze*, Per 3) [once blood is let out, relief follows instantly] and Front Valley (*Qian Gu*, SI 2).

For red facial complexion and heat coughing: Needle Branch Ditch (*Zhi Gou*, TH 6).

For copious spittle: Needle (Leg) Three *Li* (*San Li*, St 36).

Spitting and nasal running of blood is due to blood vacuity in the case of body heat. Warm blood with a hot body points to death without a remedy. (For it,) needle Hidden White (*Yin Bai*, Sp 1), Spleen *Shu* (*Pi Shu*, Bl 20), Liver *Shu* (*Gan Shu*, Bl 18), and Upper Venter (*Shang Wan*, CV 13).

---

[3] The signs and symptoms of old food malaria include belching, bad appetite, counterflow vomiting on ingestion, and abdominal fullness and distention along with alternating heat and cold. It is usually caused by retained food and contraction of external evil.

[4] Malaria mother is enduring malaria with glomus lumps in the flanks which are the result of stubborn phlegm embraced by static blood.

147

Hemafecia is governed by intestinal wind, (the problem) usually existing in the stomach and intestines. (For it,) needle Hidden White (*Yin Bai*, Sp 1) and moxa (Leg) Three *Li* (*San Li*, St 36).

In relation to the various qi (disorders), anger makes qi ascend, fright makes it chaotic, apprehension makes it descend, taxation makes it dissipate, sorrow makes it disperse, joy makes it slack, and thought makes it bind. (For these disorders:) Needle to conduct the qi.

Strangury is ascribed to heat, heat bind, inhibited phlegm qi, bladder cold *bi*, and qi vacuity in old people. (For it:) Moxa Three Yin Intersection (*San Yin Jiao*, Sp 6).

For urinary incontinence: Moxa Yang Mound Spring (*Yang Ling Quan*, GB 34) and Yin Mound Spring (*Yin Ling Quan*, Sp 9).

For throat *bi*: Needle Union Valley (*He Gu*, LI 4), Gushing Spring (*Yong Quan*, Ki 1), Celestial Chimney (*Tian Tu*, CV 22), and Bountiful Bulge (*Feng Long*, St 40). During its initial stage, moxa at the sides (of the affected place) to drain the (evil) qi.

For swelling in the head: Needle Pool at the Bend (*Qu Chi*, LI 11).

In terms of various (types of) sores:

For small and large scrofulous lumps: Moxa Shoulder Well (*Jian Jing*, GB 21), Pool at the Bend (*Qu Chi*, LI 11), and Great Reception (*Da Ying*, St 5).

For sores around the lips: Prick the lips to remove (any) malign blood.

Shan may be due to cold, qi, damp heat, or downpouring accumulated phlegm. (For it:) Needle Supreme Surge (*Tai Chong*,

Liv 3), Great Pile (*Da Dun*, Liv 1), and Severed Bone (*Jue Gu*, GB 39) and moxa Great Pile (*Da Dun*, Liv 1), Three Yin Intersection (*San Yin Jiao*, Sp 6), and the tips of the transverse crease (*i.e.*, groin) under the lower abdomen (each) with 1 cone.

Foot qi may be due to damp heat, food accumulation, (damp heat) downpouring, wind dampness, and cold dampness. (For it:) Needle Offspring of the Noble (*Gong Sun*, Sp 4) and Surging Yang (*Chong Yang*, St 42) and moxa Leg Three Li (*Zu San Li*, St 36).

Atony may be due to damp heat, phlegm, lack of blood with vacuity, qi weakness, and blood stasis. (For it:) Needle Central Metropolis (*Zhong Du*, Liv 6) and Jumping Round (*Huan Tiao*, GB 30). [It is necessary to retain the needle for 1-2 watches.] (Also) moxa (Leg) Three Li (*San Li*, St 36) and Lung *Shu* (*Fei Shu*, Bl 13).

Dyspnea is classified into phlegm dyspnea, qi vacuity, and yin vacuity (types. For it:) Moxa Central Treasury (*Zhong Fu*, Lu 1), Cloud Gate (*Yun Men*, Lu 2), Celestial Storehouse (*Tian Fu*, Lu 3), Florid Canopy (*Hua Gai*, CV 20), and Lung *Shu* (*Fei Shu*, Bl 13).

Nausea may be due to phlegm, heat, or vacuity. (For it:) Moxa Stomach *Shu* (*Wei Shu*, Bl 21), Dark Gate (*You Men*, Ki 21), Shang Hill (*Shang Qiu*, Sp 5), Central Treasury (*Zhong Fu*, Lu 1), Stone Gate (*Shi Men*, CV 5), Diaphragm *Shu* (*Ge Shu*, Bl 17), and Lumbar Yang Pass (*Yao Yang Guan*, GV 3).

Upper and lower esophageal constriction may be due to blood vacuity, qi vacuity, heat, phlegm fire, blood accumulation, and elusive mass. (For it:) Needle Celestial Chimney (*Tian Tu*, CV 22), Stone Pass (*Shi Guan*, Ki 18), (Leg) Three Li (*San Li*, St 36), Stomach *Shu* (*Wei Shu*, Bl 21), Stomach Venter (*Wei Wan*, *i.e.*, Central Venter, *Zhong Wan*, CV 12), Diaphragm *Shu* (*Ge Shu*, Bl

149

17), Water Divide (*Shui Fen*, CV 9), Sea of Qi (*Qi Hai*, CV 6), and Stomach Granary (*Wei Cang*, Bl 50).

Water swelling includes skin water, true water, stone water, and wind water.[5] It may be due to qi, dampness, and food. (For these:) Needle Stomach Granary (*Wei Cang*, Bl 50), Union Valley (*He Gu*, LI 4), Stone Gate (*Shi Men*, CV 5), Water Trough (*Shui Gou*, GV 26), (Leg) Three Li (*San Li*, St 36), Recover Flow (*Fu Liu*, Ki 7), Spring at the Bend (*Qu Quan*, Liv 8), and Fourfold Fullness (*Si Man*, Ki 14).

Inflating distention is classified into qi distention, cold distention, and spleen vacuity with central fullness (types. For it:) Needle Upper Venter (*Shang Wan*, CV 13), (Leg) Three Li (*San Li*, St 36), Screen Gate (*Zhang Men*, Liv 13), Yin Valley (*Yin Gu*, Ki 10), Origin Pass (*Guan Yuan*, CV 4), Cycle Gate (*Qi Men*, Liv 14), Moving Between (*Xing Jian*, Liv 2), Spleen *Shu* (*Pi Shu*, Bl 20), Suspended Bell (*Xuan Zhong*, GB 39), and Assuming Fullness (*Cheng Man*, St 20).

Head dizziness (is due to) qi-containing phlegm which is stirred by vacuity fire. (For it:) Needle Upper Star (*Shang Xing*, GV 23), Wind Pool (*Feng Chi*, GB 20), and Celestial Pillar (*Tian Zhu*, Bl 10).

---

[5] Skin water consists of conspicuous subcutaneous swelling all over the body which develops slowly. This is accompanied by loss of resilience of the skin, absence of sweating, no thirst, and a floating pulse. True water consists of generalized puffy swelling with abdominal fullness, dyspnea, and a deep, slow pulse. Stone water consists of hard swelling which is usually confined to the lower abdomen with distending pain in the flanks and a deep pulse. Wind water consists of swelling first appearing in the face and then developing into generalized swelling with pain in the limb joints, fever, aversion to wind, and a floating pulse.

Painful wind[6] (is due to) wind heat, wind dampness, blood vacuity, and the existence of phlegm. (For it:) Needle Hundred Convergences (*Bai Hui*, GV 20) and Jumping Round (*Huan Tiao*, GB 30).

Pain in the shoulder and upper back is mainly due to phlegm dampness. (For it:) Moxa Shoulder Bone (*Jian Yu*, LI 15) and Pool at the Bend (*Qu Chi*, LI 11).

Dream emission of essence is solely governed by intermingling of dampness and heat. (For it:) Moxa Central Pole (*Zhong Ji*, CV 3), Curved Bone (*Qu Gu*, CV 2), Gao Huang Shu (*Gao Huang Shu*, Bl 43), and Kidney *Shu* (*Shen Shu*, Bl 23).

Epilepsy is (due to) phlegm fire in all cases, and there is no need to categorize it into the six types of horse, cow, and other domesticated animals. (For it:) Moxa Hundred Convergences (*Bai Hui*, GV 20), Turtledove Tail (*Jiu Wei*, CV 15), Upper Venter (*Shang Wan*, CV 13), Spirit Gate (*Shen Men*, Ht 7), Yang Motility (*Yang Qiao*, Bl 62) [for that attacking in the day] and Yin Motility (*Yin Qiao*, Ki 6) [for that attacking in the night].

Lai[7] (is due to) contraction of ghastly killing qi between heaven and earth. That with a hoarse voice is difficult to treat. (For it:) Prick Bend Middle (*Wei Zhong*, Bl 40) to let 2-3 *he* (*i.e.*, 2-3/10 liter) of blood out. In addition, remove the malign blood from the blackish purple (venous) nodes (in the popliteal fossa).

---

6   Painful wind, a.k.a. articular wind, is painful swelling of the joints usually accompanied by restricted mobility, spontaneous sweating, fever, and, in extreme cases, swollen feet, dizziness, shortness of breath, and nausea.

7   *Lai* is leprosy.

All the above can be found in the *Za Bing Zhi Li (Illustrations of the Treatment of Miscellaneous Diseases)* by Master Liu.

Sores

(Liu) He-jian[1] said that, in connection with sores, it is necessary to determine which channel, connecting vessel, or part (is affected), how much or how little blood and qi there is, and how far or how near the points are (to the affected part before needling).

For sores breaking out on the upper back: Choose from the five points of the (foot) *tai yang*: Reaching Yin (*Zhi Yin*, Bl 67), Valley Passage (*Tong Gu*, Bl 66), Bundle Bone (*Shu Gu*, Bl 65), Kunlun (Mountain, *Kun Lun*, Bl 60), and Bend Middle (*Wei Zhong*, Bl 40).

For sores breaking out in the temporal hair: Choose from the five points of the (foot) *shao yang*: Foot Portal Yin (*Zu Qiao Yin*, GB 44), Pinched Ravine (*Xia Xi*, GB 43), Foot Overlooking Tears (*Zu Lin Qi*, GB 41), Yang Assistance (*Yang Fu*, GB 38), and Yang Mound (Spring) (*Yang Ling*, GB 34).

For sores breaking out in the moustache: Choose from the five points of the foot *yang ming*: Severe Mouth (*Li Dui*, St 45), Inner Court (*Nei Ting*, St 44), Sunken Valley (*Xian Gu*, St 43), Surging Yang (*Chong Yang*, St 42), and Ravine Divide (*Jie Xi*, St 41).

For sores breaking out in the chest: One point, Severed Bone (*Jue Gu*, GB 39)

---

[1] Liu He-jian, a.k.a. Liu Wan-su, was one of the four great masters of the Jin-Yuan dynasties. He was the founder of the School of Cool and Cold (Medicines). According to Liu, most evil qi in the body is warm or hot in nature since the host of ruling qi of the body is yang or warm.

It is said in the *Chang Yong Cuan Yao* (*Collected Essentials on Intestinal Yong*)[2] that, according to the moxa method in the *Qian Jin* (*Thousand [Pieces of] Gold*)[3], one should moxa with 100 cones at the tips of the styloid processes of the ulnae with the elbows bent. When pussy blood is precipitated, healing will occur.

It should be noted that, in terms of sores, (Liu) He-jian discussed merely the three foot yang (channels), never touching on the three hand and foot yin (channels) or the three (hand) yang (channels). Learners should extend (his discussion) by analogy (to the treatment of these other channels). In addition, a rhyme about the miscellaneous diseases in the *Yi Xue Ru Men* (*Entering the Gate of the Study of Medicine*)[4] says,

> Be careful about the (choice of) points at the initial stage of *yong* and *ju*;
> Needle the yang channels only, but never the yin ones.

These are jotted down for general reference.

---

[2] The translator fails to identify this work.

[3] *I.e.*, Sun Si-miao's *Qian Jin Yao Fang* (*Prescriptions [Worth] A Thousand [Pieces of] Gold*) written in the Tang dynasty.

[4] The *Yi Xue Ru Men* (*Entering the Gate of the Study of Medicine*) is a comprehensive medical work for beginners written by Li Yan and first published in 1575 CE.

Index

OTHER BOOKS ON CHINESE MEDICINE AVAILABLE FROM BLUE POPPY PRESS

1775 Linden Ave
Boulder, CO 80304
For ordering 1-800-487-9296
PH. 303\447-8372 FAX 303\447-0740

SEVENTY ESSENTIAL TCM FORMULAS FOR BEGINNERS by Bob Flaws, ISBN 0-936185-59-7, $19.95

CHINESE PEDIATRIC MASSAGE THERAPY: A Parent's & Practitioner's Guide to the Prevention & Treatment of Childhood Illness, by Fan Ya-li, ISBN 0-936185-54-6, $12.95

RECENT TCM RESEARCH FROM CHINA, trans. by Charles Chace & Bob Flaws, ISBN 0-936185-56-2, $18.95

EXTRA TREATISES BASED ON INVESTIGATION & INQUIRY: A Translation of Zhu Dan-xi's *Ge Zhi Yu Lun*, by Yang Shou-zhong & Duan Wu-jin, ISBN 0-936185-53-8, $15.95

A NEW AMERICAN ACUPUNCTURE by Mark Seem, ISBN 0-936185-44-9, $19.95

PATH OF PREGNANCY, VOL. I, Gestational Disorders by Bob Flaws, ISBN 0-936185-39-2, $16.95

PATH OF PREGNANCY, Vol. II, A Handbook of Traditional Chinese Postpartum Diseases by Bob Flaws. ISBN 0-936185-42-2, $18.95

HOW TO WRITE A TCM HERBAL FORMULA A Logical Methodology for the Formulation & Administration of Chinese Herbal Medicine in Decoction, by Bob Flaws, ISBN 0-936185-49-X, $10.95

FULFILLING THE ESSENCE A Handbook of Traditional & Contemporary Treatments for Female Infertility, by Bob Flaws, ISBN 0-936185-48-1, $19.95

Li Dong-yuan's TREATISE ON THE SPLEEN & STOMACH, A Translation of the *Pi Wei Lun* by Yang Shou-zhong & Li Jian-yong, ISBN 0-936185-41-4, $21.95

SCATOLOGY & THE GATE OF LIFE: The Role of the Large Intestine in Immunity by Bob Flaws ISBN 0-936185-20-1 $14.95

MENOPAUSE A Second Spring: Making a Smooth Traditiona with Traditional Chinese Medicine by Honora Lee Wolfe ISBN 0-936185-18-X $14.95

How to Have A HEALTHY PREGNANCY, HEALTHY BIRTH With Traditional Chinese Medicine by Honora Lee Wolfe, ISBN 0-936185-40-6, $9.95

MIGRAINES & TRADITIONAL CHINESE MEDICINE: A Layperson's Guide by Bob Flaws ISBN 0-936185-15-5 $11.95

STICKING TO THE POINT: A Rational Methodology for the Step by Step Formulation & Administration of an Acupuncture Treatment by Bob Flaws ISBN 0-936185-17-1 $14.95

ENDOMETRIOSIS, INFERTILITY AND TRADITIONAL CHINESE MEDICINE: A Laywoman's Guide by Bob Flaws ISBN 0-936185-14-7 $9.95

THE BREAST CONNECTION: A Laywoman's Guide to the Treatment of Breast Disease by Chinese Medicine by Honora Lee Wolfe ISBN 0-936185-13-9 $9.95

NINE OUNCES: A Nine Part Program For The Prevention of AIDS in HIV Positive Persons by Bob Flaws ISBN 0-936185-12-0 $9.95

THE TREATMENT OF CANCER BY INTEGRATED CHINESE-WESTERN MEDICINE by Zhang Dai-zhao, trans. by Zhang Ting-liang & Bob Flaws, ISBN 0-936185-11-2 $18.95

A HANDBOOK OF TRADITIONAL CHINESE DERMATOLOGY by Liang Jian-hui, trans. by Zhang Ting-liang & Bob Flaws, ISBN 0-936185-07-4 $15.95

A HANDBOOK OF TRADITIONAL CHINESE GYNECOLOGY by Zhejiang College of TCM, trans. by Zhang Ting-liang, ISBN 0-936185-06-6 (2nd edit.) $21.95

PRINCE WEN HUI'S COOK: Chinese Dietary Therapy by Bob Flaws & Honora Lee Wolfe, ISBN 0-912111-05-4, $12.95 (Published by Paradigm Press, Brookline, MA)

THE DAO OF INCREASING LONGEVITY AND CONSERVING ONE'S LIFE by Anna Lin & Bob Flaws, ISBN 0-936185-24-4 $16.95

FIRE IN THE VALLEY: The TCM Diagnosis and Treatment of Vaginal Diseases by Bob Flaws ISBN 0-936185-25-2 $16.95

HIGHLIGHTS OF ANCIENT ACUPUNCTURE PRESCRIPTIONS trans. by Honora Lee Wolfe & Rose Crescenz ISBN 0-936185-23-6 $14.95

ARISAL OF THE CLEAR: A Simple Guide to Healthy Eating According to Traditional Chinese Medicine by Bob Flaws, ISBN #-936185-27-9 $8.95

PEDIATRIC BRONCHITIS: Its Cause, Diagnosis & Treatment According to Traditional Chinese Medicine trans. by Gao Yu-li and Bob Flaws, ISBN 0-936185-26-0 $15.95

AIDS & ITS TREATMENT ACCORDING TO TRADITIONAL CHINESE MEDICINE by Huang Bing-shan, trans. by Fu-Di & Bob Flaws, ISBN 0-936185-28-7 $24.95

ACUTE ABDOMINAL SYNDROMES: Their Diagnosis & Treatment by Combined Chinese-Western Medicine by Alon Marcus, ISBN 0-936185-31-7 $16.95

MY SISTER, THE MOON: The Diagnosis & Treatment of Menstrual Diseases by Traditional Chinese Medicine by Bob Flaws, ISBN 0-936185-34-1, $24.95

FU QING-ZHU'S GYNECOLOGY trans. by Yang Shou-zhong and Liu Da-wei, ISBN 0-936185-35-X, $21.95

FLESHING OUT THE BONES: The Importance of Case Histories in Chinese Medicine trans. by Charles Chace. ISBN 0-936185-30-9, $18.95

CLASSICAL MOXIBUSTION SKILLS in Contemporary Clinical Practice by Sung Baek, ISBN 0-936185-16-3 $10.95

THE MEDICAL I CHING: Oracle of the Healer Within by Miki Shima, OMD, ISBN 0-936185-38-4, $19.95

MASTER TONG'S ACUPUNCTURE: An Ancient Lineage for Modern Practice, trans. and commentary by Miriam Lee, OMD, ISBN 0-936185-37-6, $19.95

A HANDBOOK OF TCM UROLOGY & MALE SEXUAL DYSFUNCTION by Anna Lin, OMD, ISBN 0-936185-36-8, $16.95

PMS: Its Cause, Diagnosis & Treatment According to Traditional Chinese Medicine by Bob Flaws ISBN 0-936185-22-8 $14.95

MASTER HUA'S CLASSIC OF THE CENTRAL VISCERA by Hua Tuo, ISBN 0-936185-43-0, $21.95

THE HEART & ESSENCE OF DAN-XI'S METHODS OF TREATMENT by Xu Dan-xi, trans. by Yang Shou-zhong, ISBN 0-926185-49-X, $21.95

STATEMENTS OF FACT IN TRADITIONAL CHINESE MEDICINE by Bob Flaws, ISBN 0-936185-52-X, $10.95

IMPERIAL SECRETS OF HEALTH & LONGEVITY by Bob Flaws, ISBN 0-936185-51-1, $9.95

THE SYSTEMATIC CLASSIC OF ACUPUNCTURE & MOXIBUSTION (*Jia Yi Jing*) by Huang-fu Mi, trans. by Yang Shou-zhong and Charles Chace, ISBN 0-936185-29-5, $79.95